Yourfitnesssuccess.com

Yoga For Strength And Stability

Progressive yoga poses for senior fitness, Beginners and Beyond

James Atkinson

Copyright ©

2025 yourfitnesssuccess.com

All rights reserved

Contents

Introduction 1
Health Check 4
The foundations of physical yoga 5
What you will need 8
Breathing 10
Alignment and control 13
Starting positions 18
Entering a yoga pose 33
The poses 36
Tree Pose 37
Warrior 44
Eagle 49
Dancer 56
Chair 63
Four-Limbed Staff Pose 69
Bridge pose 72
Forward fold 75
Cobra 81
Happy baby 85
Goddess pose 88
Roll down 94
Putting it all together 98
Chair yoga poses 112
Your yoga routine 126
Video course 127
Blank routine cards 130

Also by James Atkinson 137

Introduction

Welcome to your yoga journey! At the heart of this guide, there is a focus on longevity and physical function for everyone. 10 – 15 minutes of daily yoga exercise can make a significant positive change to anyone's physical and mental condition. Whether you are a twenty-year-old athlete or a senior fitness beginner, we can all benefit from yoga.

The art of yoga and its history is extremely involved, and there's a lot to it. But this guide focuses on the physical aspect of yoga to develop longevity and function throughout the whole body. Although physical development is the primary goal, if performed correctly and consistently, other benefits commonly associated with yoga will develop as positive side effects.

Mindfulness is needed to engage specific muscle groups and maintain concentration. Controlled breathing also enhances focus and can lower stress levels. Whilst many other exercise forms also offer these benefits, yoga gives us a greater opportunity to train our mind and body simultaneously.

The development of full body strength, flexibility, stability and balance for everyday activities is something that everyone can engage in to enhance, or even drastically improve, their quality of life. A regular yoga routine designed with this in mind is the perfect solution. No age limits, low physical barrier to entry, low-impact exercise, minimal to no equipment, no gym memberships, short workouts. Yoga will truly benefit anyone interested in physical development.

So, for this guide, we focus on the following pillars:

Strength

Flexibility

Stability

Balance

Although many yoga poses and flows offer the development of all these pillars of fitness, some poses may prioritise one or more over the others. For example, a yoga pose may challenge our balance as a priority, meaning we will develop balance along with muscle strength in the engaged muscle groups.

For this guide, yoga poses used in the flows and illustrations, there is an overlap in as many of the pillars as possible to give well-rounded physical exercise sessions.

I'm Jim from yourfitnesssuccess.com. A qualified fitness instructor with a military background that's been involved in fitness for most of my life, long distance running, endurance training and bodybuilding. Lifting weights in the gym and resistance training has always been my constant, however.

Before I had earned any formal fitness qualifications, I lifted weights regularly, just like many guys in their late teens and early twenties did in the late 90s / early 2000s. Arnold Schwarzenegger and Sylvester Stallone have a lot to answer to!

It became part of my life and I got to the point where I wanted to be better, so after a stint in the military, part of adjusting to civilian life was to find a civilian job. The obvious move for me was to do something in the fitness industry, but I wanted more knowledge on bodybuilding for my personal goals. The search began for a fitness qualification company that specialised in this. The organisation I landed on was WABBA which was linked to an amazing bodybuilder called Serge Nubret. This was more than good enough for me!

I learned a tremendous amount from the guys at WABBA. It changed my perspective and entire mind-set for exercise and fitness forever. One of the big revelations, if not the biggest, was the "mind and muscle" connection. In simple terms; if you are performing a bicep curl, you are training your bicep for optimal development. If you can feel this muscle working to its maximum contraction and full extension, you are doing it right. If not, consider reassessing your exercise form or resistance level.

Why is this brief back story relevant to yoga? Since gaining formal qualifications with WABBA and practicing what I had learned, prioritising the "mind / muscle" connection along with using correct exercise form has been the number one fundamental element in all aspects of fitness that I practice and advise in. This fundamental factor fits perfectly with yoga.

During the evolution of my own fitness endeavours, I've seen increasing value in yoga training, almost to the point it is a necessity or, at worse, an extremely valuable tool that can be used to enhance other fitness goals. So whether you are a total beginner to fitness, a senior trainer or a seasoned fitness veteran, you will benefit from yoga training. Let's get into it!

Health Check

Before you embark on any fitness routine, please consult your doctor or physiotherapist. If you have any health conditions, always check if the type of exercise and exercise choices you intend to involve yourself with.

1. Do not exercise if you are unwell.

2. Stop if you feel pain, and if the pain does not subside, consult your doctor or physiotherapist.

3. Do not exercise if you have taken alcohol or had a large meal in the last few hours.

4. If you are taking medication, please check with your doctor to make sure it is okay for you to exercise.

5. If in doubt at all, please check with your doctor or physiotherapist first – you may even want to take this routine and go through it with them. It may be helpful to ask for a blood pressure, cholesterol and weight check. You can then have these taken again in a few months to see the benefit.

The foundations of physical yoga

I've always been of the opinion that the more we know about why we are doing what we are doing in exercise helps with development in a big way. Understanding the reason for any exercise movement not only increases our ability to perform it correctly, but it offers us the knowledge and opportunity to adapt the movement to ensure we get the most out of it, making each exercise session more effective.

In some of my other resistance and weight training guides, there is more than a simple nod to different types of exercises for different types of fitness goals. If we follow these guides, we would know the difference between a compound exercise, an isolation exercise, and when and why we'd use each of these in our workouts.

In this sense, Yoga is no different. Although this guide is set up to encompass five pillars of fitness and focus on well-rounded physical workouts, it's true to say that knowing why we are doing what we are doing is not as important here. This is assuming that we follow this guide and not take yoga any further. For some people, this is just fine.

But I highly recommend that from the start, you make a conscious effort to understand which muscle groups and range of movements are engaged in each pose or movement. You make a mind muscle connection and focus on the exercise form as a priority. In any exercise method, correct exercises form should be the foundation. If you feel that a certain pose or movement is awkward or uncomfortable, find a mirror or record yourself performing it. You can study your alignment, posture, and exercise form this way. It's always worth taking the time to do this.

The understanding of function for each pose and movement is developed over time while we are training. It's a practical skill that we can always improve on if we are conscious of our exercise form and the muscle groups involved in the movements. If the correct exercise form is the foundation, the five pillars of fitness that this guide sets out to develop can be seen as the training effect of performing these movements, consistently and over time. Let's look at these in more detail.

Strength

Strength in yoga, and for the purpose of this guide, is the conditioning of a muscle group to develop the ability to hold a position by engaging for greater periods or performing more repetitions of a movement. Strength development in our abdominal and lower back muscles plays a big part in yoga and in this sense. Strength has an overlap with stability and balance.

Flexibility

Flexibility is the range of motion of our joints. Every joint in our body has a specific functional design. For example; Knees and elbows bend, hips and shoulders rotate. The development of flexibility is to condition joints to be able to achieve a full range of motion without experiencing pain. Generally speaking, working on flexibility by moving through full range of motion will develop function in the muscles associated with the movement.

Stability

The meaning of stability in this guide is the ability to build a position or pose under control and to hold the pose in a stable manner. Moving in and out of a yoga pose under control and with confidence will challenge every stabiliser muscle in the engaged groups through their full range of motion. With a focus on stability and controlled movements, muscle groups will adapt and engage during all types of everyday activities and give confidence in movement. Stability has some crossover with balance.

Balance

Balance has a twofold meaning in this particular yoga guide. The ability to perform exercises that include certain movements, like standing on one leg comfortably, is the obvious one. The more we perform balancing exercises, the better our stability will become. The second meaning to balance is the balancing of muscle groups by challenging them all with strength, flexibility, stability and balancing exercises equally.

As strength, flexibility, stability and balance in our muscles develop, the exercise or movement will become more comfortable, flow better and be more fulfilling to perform. Seeing progress in any fitness venture is very rewarding, and yoga happens to be a fitness method that garners fast results, especially for the beginner.

What you will need

You don't need a lot of equipment to practise yoga, a small space that you can stretch out in, and yourself. There is, however, yoga equipment widely available that can help you out during your sessions.

Although it's not a necessity, some yoga equipment may help you with better comfort, stability and security with your sessions. There may be some specific situations where an individual struggling with a progression can use these aids to help them to the next level.

I wouldn't advise anyone to go out and collect all the pieces of yoga equipment available before starting, except maybe a yoga mat or socks if they are planning to practise yoga on a slippery floor. But it's worth knowing about them in case the need arises later on.

Practicing yoga with bare feet on the grass or sand can connect us to nature. It can be grounding and sensory, which compliments some traditional core values of yoga, such as mindfulness and harmony. However, in a practical sense, there are some potential issues, especially for the beginner. Uneven ground and varying resistance levels under foot can change our position and put undue strain on some joints. The ideal surface should be flat, even, firm and non-slip.

A room with a fixed carpet will do the job nicely. If you have a tiled or laminated type floor, it may be a good idea to invest in a yoga mat. Yoga socks are not as optimal as a mat, as they are less stable. From a practical view, barefoot on a yoga mat placed on a firm, even, flat floor, in a room or outside space is a great option.

When progressing through the stages of a yoga pose, you may feel the need for support if you need to balance. Having a support to steady yourself so you can hold a pose can be an excellent way to hold a position without having to reset. A sturdy chair or wall is great for this. Not to be used as a crutch, this is more for assurance to gently steady yourself if you need it. There are some exercises in this guide that illustrate this option.

Some variations of yoga pose may require additional support for individuals. If, for example, you feel uncomfortable kneeling or lying on a mat; it is entirely acceptable to use a kneeling pad, rolled-up towel or other form of cushioning placed on your contact point of discomfort. If you do opt for such a thing, it's best to make sure the cushion is even and a nonslip material.

Breathing

Breathing is involuntary for most of us, so it's an action that is taken for granted, but the act of breathing is one of the fundamental conditions of life. This translates to the art of yoga in that every yoga movement starts with a deliberate breathing technique. From a physical standpoint, we can stabilise our exercise form and prepare for movement on exhalation. Core strength and stability are beneficial for everybody, but learning to control breathing is where yoga really begins.

Correct breathing techniques can lead to better focus and mindfulness. If we are concentrating on breathing whilst performing yoga exercise, we leave behind other thoughts and stresses from everyday life. This has a positive impact on our nervous system; once we find our rhythm, our parasympathetic nervous system activates, which lowers stress levels, slows our heart rate and promotes relaxation.

There are many breathing techniques used in yoga. To cover these in depth would warrant a full standalone guide, but we will focus on two forms that can be used on their own or in conjunction with yoga exercise.

Diaphragmatic breathing is a form of breathing that can be used during exercise, meditation, or to reduce stress. As this is a foundation skill that will enhance our yoga sessions significantly, we can practise this before we even think about performing any yoga pose. Consider this an exercise in itself. I would go as far as saying that diaphragmatic breathing is the gateway to starting yoga.

Diaphragmatic breathing:

1. Lie on a mat or sit on a chair with a straight back
2. Place one hand on your stomach and the other on your chest
3. Inhale slowly until you feel your stomach expand
4. Continue the inhalation until your chest expands
5. Once your lungs are about 80-90 per cent full, slowly exhale
6. Your chest will return to the start position and then your stomach
7. Continue the exhalation until your abdomen muscles naturally engage
8. Repeat until you have a steady, natural breathing rhythm going

The above breathing process is a foundation yoga breathing style, also known as "belly breathing". This can be performed as a standalone exercise whilst lying flat on our back, sitting on a chair with a flat back, and once this technique is familiar, during yoga poses and movements, too. This form of breathing is an excellent way to release stress, promote relaxation, and focus. We could all use this exercise now and then so, I'd advise taking some time to become familiar with this breathing exercise. You can give it a go right now!

Looking at this breathing technique from a more physical aspect, and in order to develop core stability, there are a few tweaks we can make to this exercise. This next technique is still a yoga practice, but it is normally used in dynamic yoga exercise for stability and to strengthen the core muscles.

If you are a beginner, I would advise that you become comfortable with diaphragmatic breathing before using the abdominal lock technique whilst exercising. Using the abdominal lock technique adds an extra variable to our workouts, while there is already a lot to concentrate on, so this may cause overwhelm or undue fatigue for some.

Abdominal lock breathing:

1. Exhale slowly emptying your lungs until you feel your abdomen muscles naturally engage
2. Before you inhale again, actively take control of your abdomen muscles that have just engaged, keeping them contracted
3. As you inhale, you will now feel your chest expand
4. Exhale again, keeping your abdominals engaged
5. Repeat until you have a steady, natural breathing rhythm going

This method of breathing also takes some practice. It may feel unnatural at first, but it is surprising how quickly this can change with a bit of consistency. Although this breathing style has more physical benefits to muscle development, it also promotes mind and muscle connection, as we are actively singling out our transverse abdominal muscles with the continued engagement. As mentioned, the abdominal lock breathing technique may not be ideal for beginners, but by using it as a separate exercise for familiarity and foundational conditioning of the abdominals, we can look towards adding this to our workouts as a progression step.

For beginners, breathing techniques can be challenging to master, especially when trying to position the body correctly throughout yoga movements. A great way to develop these techniques is to incorporate them into a beginner routine coupled with the start positions. This way, we are developing two foundational practices simultaneously and potentially relieving stress levels. There is a routine card for this later in the guide for more clarity to either follow exactly, or tweak according to your specific needs.

Alignment and control

Like breathing in yoga, alignment is another dense topic as it leans heavily into biomechanics. The deeper the understanding of movement, muscular synergy and muscle function throughout the human body, the better we can apply exercise in any form, not just yoga. But this yoga book aims to distil these subjects into manageable, easy to digest information, highlighting what we need to get started and to progress.

First, let's look at a real life example of movement to highlight the general principals of alignment when practicing yoga.

During my personal training days, to demonstrate the importance of correct exercise form, and the importance of consciously targeting muscle groups for my clients in their upcoming gym sessions, I would ask them to stand on one leg by aiming to bring the upper part of the lifted leg (quadriceps) to as parallel to the floor as possible.

This test fits very nicely with the concept of alignment in yoga and "the importance of correct exercise form, and the importance of consciously targeting muscle groups" in general resistance training terms translates to the correct alignment, control and mindful movement in yoga terms.

This type of thing was a very common response:

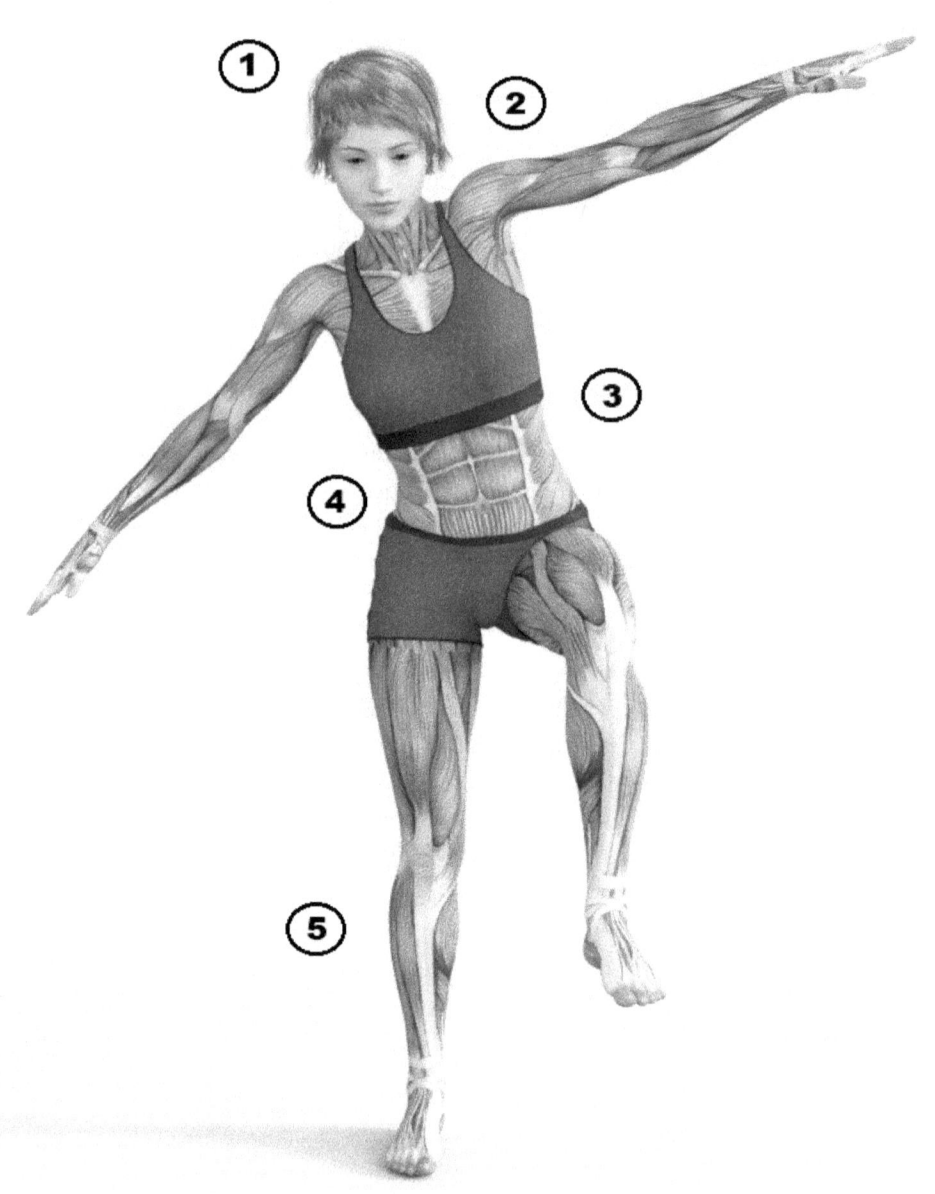

1. Head tilted, taking alignment from the spine
2. Shoulder raised on the leg lift side and arms offset
3. Upper body shifted to the balancing leg side, taking further alignment from the spine
4. Hips hinging forward slightly and to the balancing side
5. Knee locked diluting engagement in the balancing quadriceps and weight distribution shifted to the outside leg, causing uneven distribution of pressure on the knee

This may seem very critical, but the truth is, anyone who doesn't have interest in fitness, biomechanics and mindful movement can be forgiven as the request was to "stand on one leg". So, in a sense, this is a job well done!

If we are mindful of our movement, muscular control, and aim for correct alignment before attempting to stand on one leg, we would get something like this:

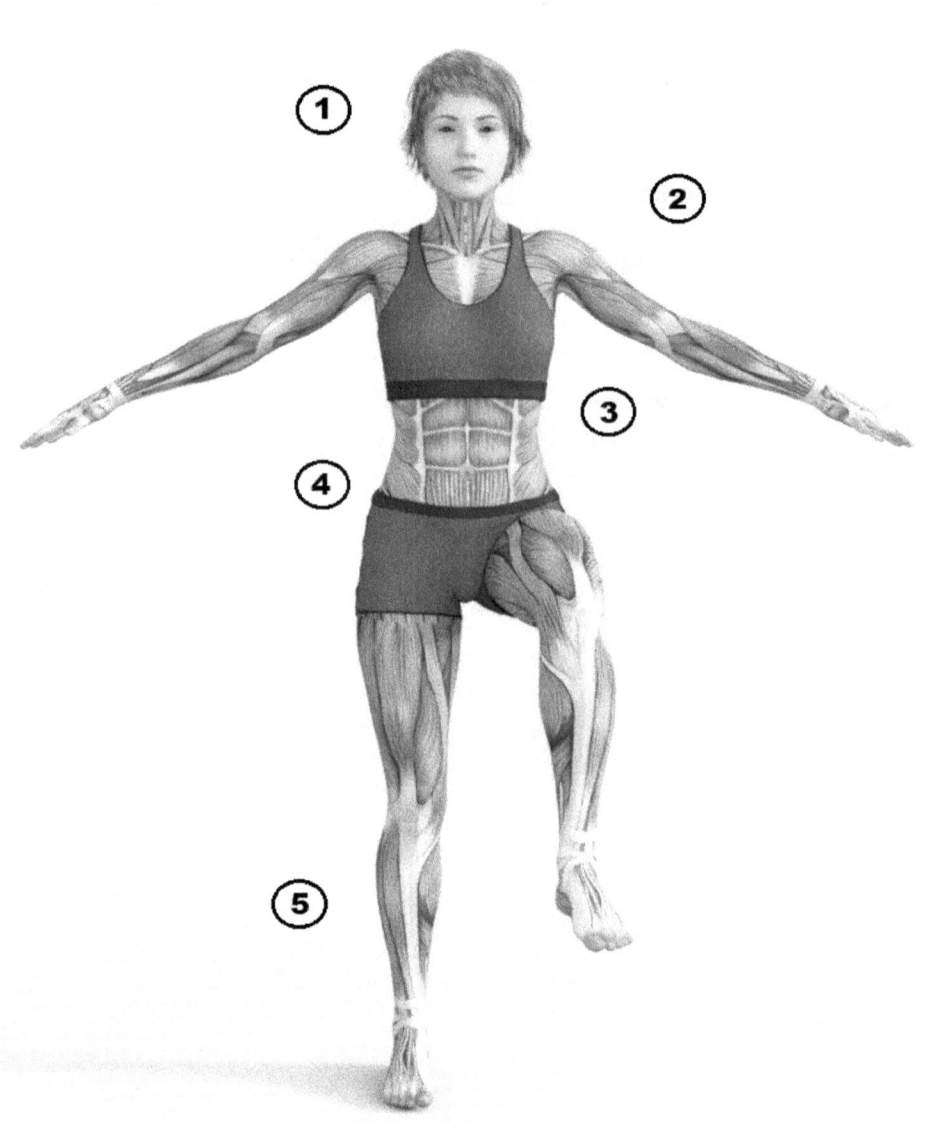

1. Head and neck in a neutral position, aligning the top of the spine
2. Shoulders and arms mirroring each other
3. Torso remains central in all planes of movement, aligning the mid to lower spine
4. Hips parallel to the ground, aligning the lower spine and engaging appropriate muscle groups for the movement
5. Knee slightly bent, and body weight distributed evenly through the sole of the foot

The difference between the two illustrations is fairly stark in places and fairly subtle in others.

To sum up the first illustration: Standing on one leg using balance and shifting body weight in order to complete the task.

To sum up the second illustration: Standing on one leg with a focus on alignment, mindful muscle movement and muscular control.

Performing this task as per the second illustration is a lot more challenging due to the structured mindful approach and physical element. We must:

- Prepare for the movement by controlling our breathing
- Engage our core muscles as we shift our bodyweight evenly to the planted foot
- Ensure our alignment stays neutral in all planes as we lift our opposite foot from the ground
- Control muscle groups in the legs, core, back and shoulders throughout the movement to maintain correct form
- Maintain our breathing rhythm and be mindful of our alignment throughout the movement

Some may say that standing on one leg is a simple task, and for many, it is, but to stand on one leg using mindful muscular control, alignment, and grace makes the task an aspirational one.

Attaining the ability to reach good alignment and muscular control to perform advanced yoga poses is all part of the development, and this comes with consistent training and practice. So it's extremely important that we never sacrifice alignment and exercise form in order to progress in a pose.

Starting positions

Yoga exercise encourages us to twist, bend, rotate, extend and flex. The goal is typically to maintain or return to neutral alignment, to ensure safety and stability. With every twist, bend and extension, these dynamic movements challenge our strength, flexibility, and balance, but we begin with a critical foundation.

The starting position for any yoga pose is very important. It's from this position that we build and develop the movement through all variants and stages of the pose. The starting position is a physical necessity that gives us a solid foundation to work from, but we can also use this opportunity to mentally prepare and plan for movement.

Yoga poses are not restricted to a single start position as we can perform them from a seated, standing, prone, four point contact, or supine position. For every start position, however, we can apply some general rules to each of these. These rules are focused on alignment and correct positioning of the back, spine and hips in order to maintain spinal integrity and stability.

Transverse alignment: "Twisting"

The transverse plane divides the body into upper and lower halves. Use this to avoid unintended twists. At the start of a movement, we should aim to maintain alignment in this plane by ensuring we are not twisting at the hips or through the back and shoulders. Neutral alignment in this plane ensures our spine is not rotated or twisted at the start of a yoga pose.

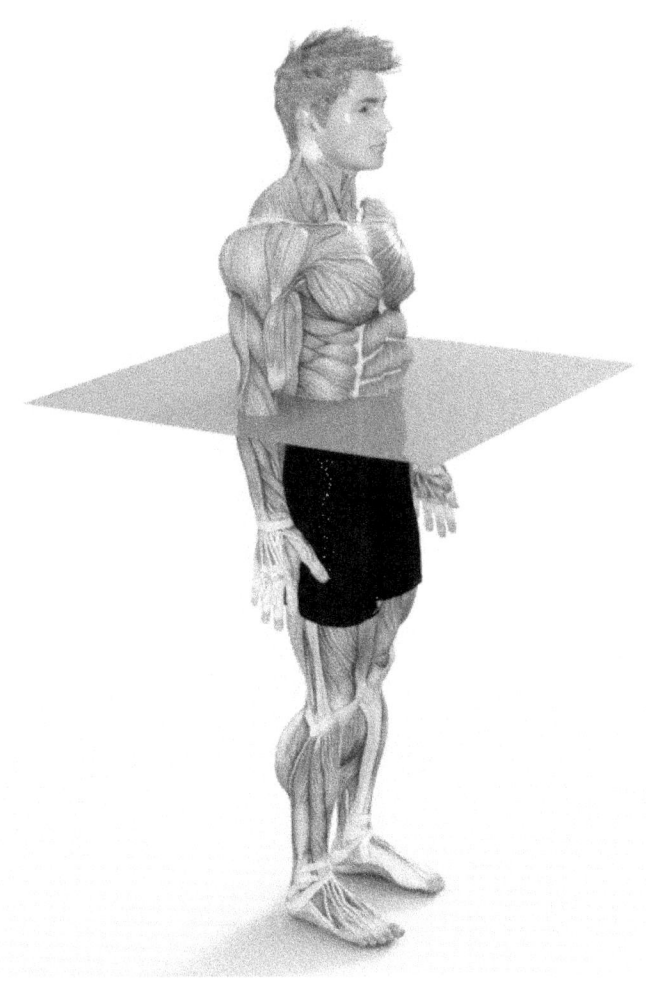

Sagittal alignment: "Bending forward or backwards"

The sagittal plane divides the body into right and left halves. Use this to avoid excessive flexion or extension. At the start of the movement, we should ensure that our spine is neutral on this plane. By keeping neutral from front to back, we should not be leaning forward, arching our backs (hyper extending) and shoulders should not be rolled forward.

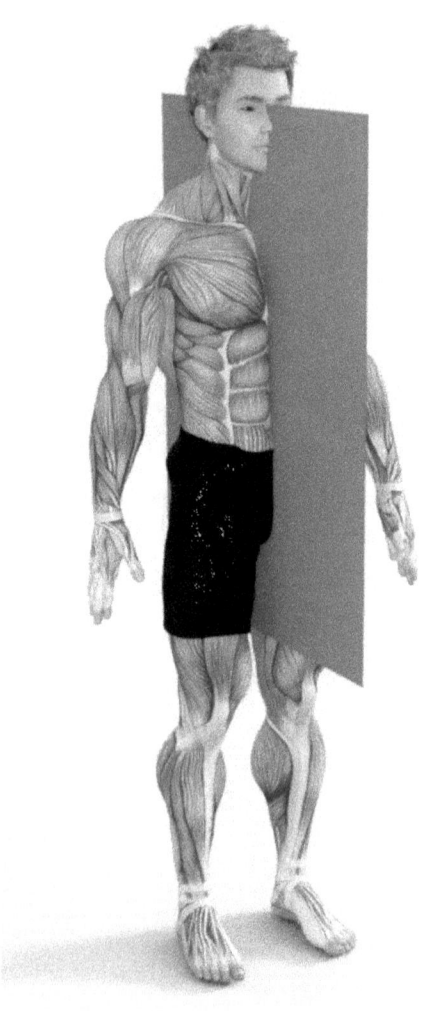

Frontal plane: "Side to side"

The frontal plane divides the body into front and back. Use this to prevent lateral tilt. At the start of a yoga pose, we should make sure to align in this plane by even weight distribution through our ground contact points through both sides of our bodies, ensuring we are not leaning more to the left or right.

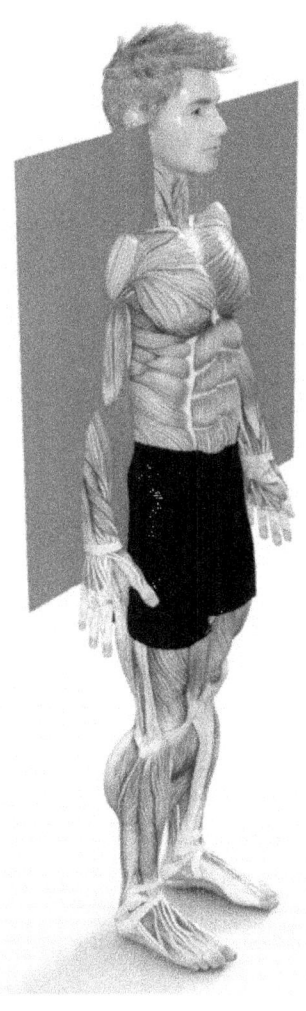

Once in the start position, we can start our breathing techniques and engage our core. Before moving into any variation of a pose, we can take some time to think about our alignment, our breathing and the next steps towards movement we are going to take. On returning to the start position, it's a good idea to "reset", think about our alignment again, control our breathing and prepare our minds for the next movement.

Starting positions for seated, standing, lying and four point contact are shown below. For total beginners, planning a yoga session can be composed exclusively of these static positions. If you feel this might be for you, this is what I would advise:

- Plan to hold each position for 1 to 2 minutes
- Whilst in the position, think about your alignment on all planes and make adjustments as needed
- Be mindful of weight distribution. Ensure that it's always evenly distributed through your contact points
- Concentrate on your breathing whilst engaging your core muscles on the exhale
- When you become confident in these positions, as a progression, you could try "abdominal lock" breathing

When practicing the following starting positions, keep in mind the alignment principals discussed. Whilst in these positions, think about your movement in each of the planes and adjust accordingly. You can work from your lower body to your upper body, checking off as you go:

- Is my weight distributed evenly through my contact points?
- Are my hips tilted or twisted?
- Is my lower back flat?
- Are my shoulders sagging forward?
- Is my head in a neutral position?
- Is my breathing as it should be?

With enough practice, this will become second nature and feel very natural.

Chair yoga starting position

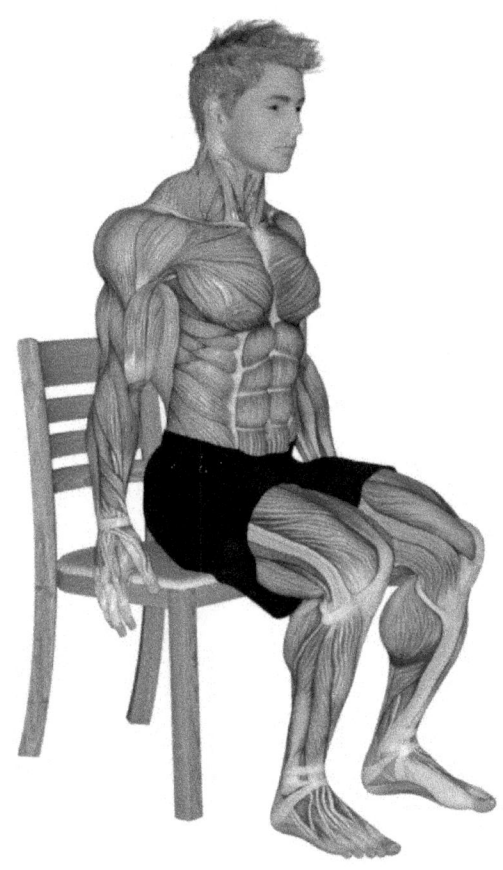

- Choose a sturdy, flat chair or stool without wheels
- Sit upright, with your body weight evenly distributed across your left and right glutes (sit bones)
- Your feet should be flat on the floor in line with your hips and knees
- Knees should be bent to form an angle of about 90 degrees between your calfs a hamstrings
- Rest your arms by your sides a keep your head in a neutral position

This starting position for seated yoga is excellent for the beginner. It's also great for breathing practice and relaxation purposes as it's considered more comfortable that other starting position variations for most.

When choosing a chair for seated yoga, some consider a high, straight back rather than a stool or bench. Although the back of the chair is not used for direct support in this position, this is for those who would like extra insurance. Knowing you have a support behind you if you need it can promote confidence.

Standing starting position

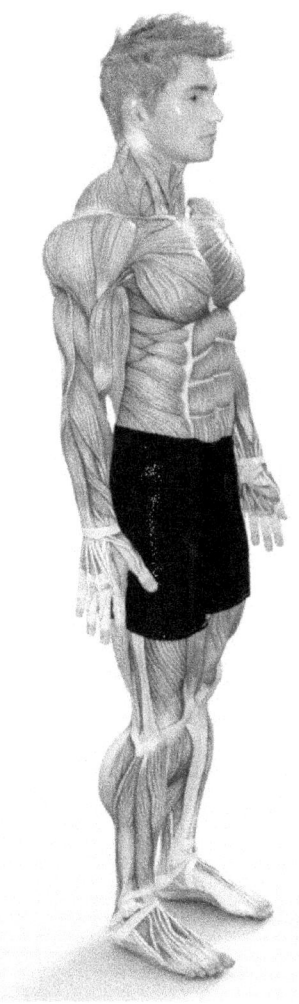

- Stand with your feet flat on the floor about hip width apart
- Legs should be straight but with a slight bend in the knees to engage the quads
- Arms should be relaxed by your sides, palms facing inwards
- Head in a neutral position, looking forward

This variation of a standing start position is great for the beginner as it gives the opportunity to practice mindfulness, muscle awareness, general alignment principals and even weight distribution through the contact points (feet).

It is common to move the feet together so the big toes and heels are in contact with each other, but this may reduce stability and balance for some people.

Seated on floor starting position

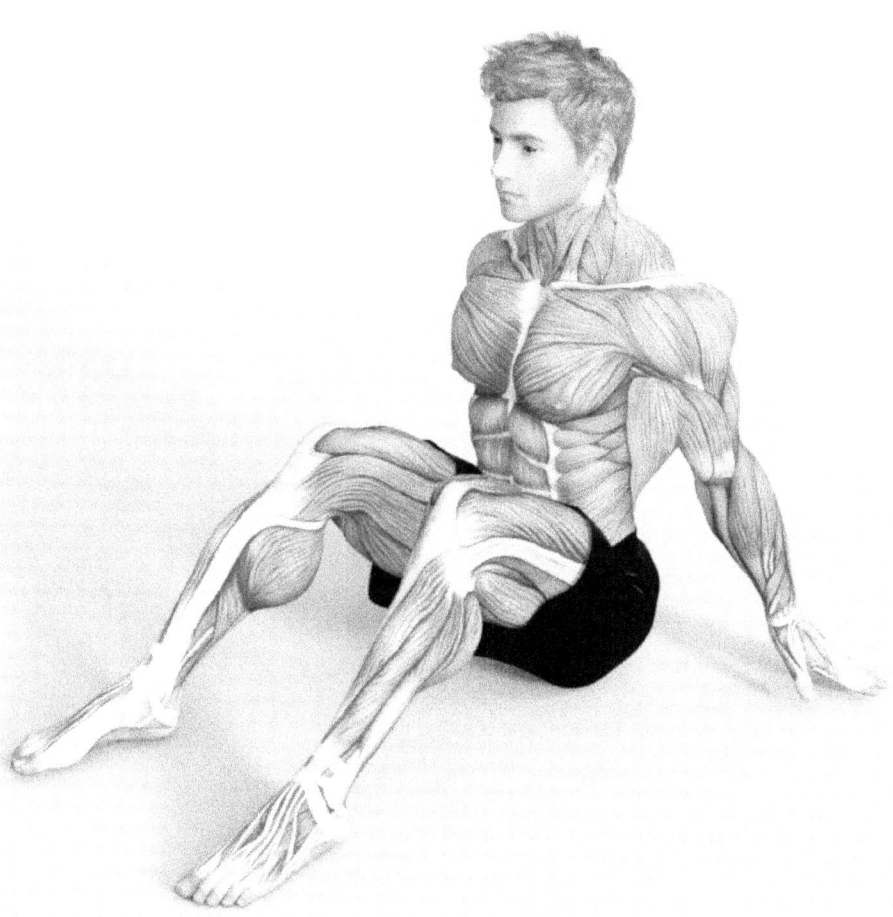

- Sit on the floor with your knees bent and feet in full contact with the ground
- Back should be flat and head in a neutral position
- Pull your arms backwards slightly and to your sides
- Steady yourself by making light contact with the ground with your fingertips

- Your feet, sit bones and fingertips should be in contact with the ground

This seated starting position is useful for those who are unfamiliar with floor exercises in general. Sitting in this position gives us the opportunity to engage our core muscles with control. If we hinge forward at the hips slightly to transfer our body weight from our fingertips and onto our sit bones, the core is challenged further. This is a great way for beginners to familiarise core engagement.

Ideally, our feet should be about hip width apart, but they can be placed in a wider position if stability is an issue. The narrower the feet and knee position, the more challenging this position becomes.

Four point starting position

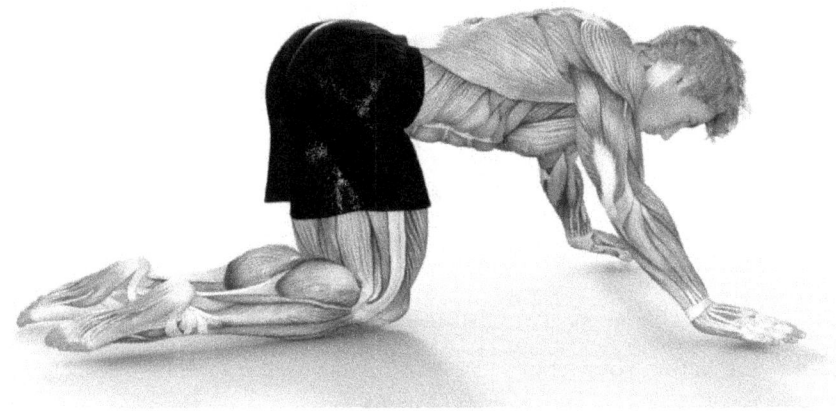

- From a kneeling position, hinge at the hips to bring the upper body parallel to the ground
- As you move into this position, bring your arms forward to support your bodyweight. Palms should be flat on the ground directly under your shoulders
- Knees should be directly beneath your hips and hip width apart
- The fronts of your lower legs and feet should be in contact with the ground

This is a starting position for several poses, but there are some modifications that can be made depending on comfort and mobility. Rather than placing the hands directly beneath the shoulders, some people use the mid chest. This can shift bodyweight forward slightly, engaging the core and shoulders more, but it can put more stress on the wrists for some.

Prone starting position

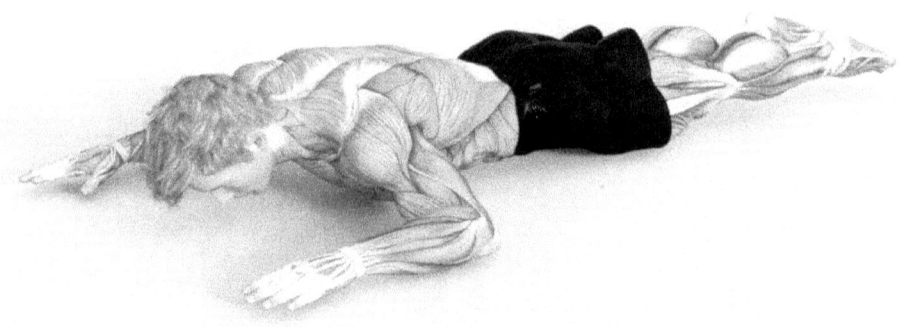

- Lie flat on your front
- Feet and knees should be hip width apart and toes should be pointed back
- Position your arms so your palms are flat on the ground in line with your head by bending at the elbows
- Rest your forehead on the ground and apply a small amount of pressure through your palms so your bodyweight is not concentrated through your forehead

This version of a prone starting position is great for the beginner and for those who have tension in the neck, as resting the forehead on the ground helps with neutral neck alignment and reduces muscle engagement in the neck.

Supine starting position

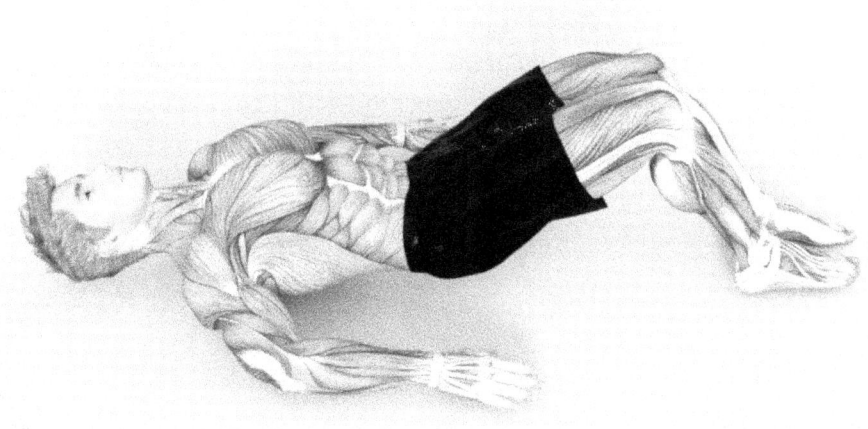

- Sit on the floor and slowly roll back so your upper glutes and lower back make contact with the floor
- Continue this roll back through your middle to upper back and through your shoulders until the rear of your head is resting on the floor
- Bring your arms to your sides, palms down and in contact with the ground
- Pull your knees towards your chest until the soles of your feet are in contact with the ground

This version of a supine starting position is great for the beginner, those with tight hamstrings or lower back issues. Raising the knees and planting the soles of the feet on the ground aids in alignment of the lower back. Another option for a supine starting position is to straighten the legs so their rear and heals of the feet make contact with the ground. This may be uncomfortable for some, however.

To sum up

We should begin every yoga pose by establishing a neutral spine in the sagittal plane (avoiding excessive flexion or extension), ensuring symmetry and even weight distribution in the frontal plane (preventing lateral tilt), and maintaining a stable, non-rotated position in the transverse plane (avoiding unintended twists). Engage the core and ground evenly through the body's contact points to support alignment across all planes.

Entering a yoga pose

Every yoga pose we perform requires us to go through a certain sequence. It may be helpful to look at this sequence as "building the pose". Although yoga poses can be performed standing, seated, on all fours, or lying, the same process can be used in all forms.

Before each session, ideally, we should have a plan. This should include the poses we are going to use, for how long and in which order. More on this later, but once this is in place, we can use the following process when entering each pose:

Breathing and posture

Prepare by getting into the appropriate start position for the planned yoga pose, whether this is standing, seated, prone, four point contact, or supine position. Make sure to practise the principals of alignment and posture from the previous chapters as you do this. Once in position, take some time to breathe and focus. There is no rush to start moving. At this point, think about your breathing rhythm. Aim for steady, intentional breaths to feel your chest rise on inhalation and stomach muscles engage on exhalation.

Neutral posture and alignment

Once breathing rhythm is established we should reassess neutral position and alignment. Although posture and alignment is practiced when entering the start position, we should reassess before movement. Sometimes, for beginners especially, breathing with intention and the concentration that it requires can have an effect on our alignment. So before movement, we check our alignment is good; contact points are evenly grounded, hips central, spine is aligned in all planes, shoulders are not hunched and head is in a neutral position.

Movement

Once breathing is established, alignment and posture have been checked, it's time to move. Before you start any movement, take some time to visualise what you would like to do; How will the movement affect your alignment and which muscles will you have to engage to keep it as it should be? Once you are ready, begin the movement in synergy with your breath. Typically, inhale during movements that lengthen, expand, or open the body, such as lifting arms overhead, arching the back, or extending into poses. We should typically exhale during movements that contract, deepen, or stabilise, such as folding forward, twisting, or bending.

When moving from one position to the next, focus on steady, controlled motion. If you need to pause to adjust balance or alignment part way through a movement, do so. This can help to develop muscle strength, awareness, and mindfulness.

On reaching the planned progression point of a pose, hold for your planned time or breath count before returning to the start position.

Progression

Each yoga pose in this guide has a set of progressions, each depicted by a single illustration. The first progression for any pose is the starting position. Once this is achievable, we can move onto the next and so on. You can choose how far you wish to progress in each pose based on your goals and physical ability.

If you do wish to try a new progression that challenges your skill, before returning to the start position after your current limit, test the next progression out for several seconds or breaths. If you are comfortable, able to maintain alignment, balance and breathing, you can increase the time spent on this next time round. Eventually, this will become your first movement phase from the start position.

It's extremely important to note, however, that you should never sacrifice form, stability, breathing rhythm, or alignment to transition from one progression to the next. If you find yourself struggling with this, you can either spend more time practicing at your current level or try to find a position between the progression step, where you are stable and comfortable, and work in smaller movement increments from here.

To sum up

For beginners to yoga, applying these steps to the first progression of any given yoga pose in this guide, or even following them to enter a start position, can set a great foundation for progress. It may, however, be slightly overwhelming for some. If you find this is the case, try to work on one aspect at a time and remember the process as: "breathe, align, move, hold".

If you wish to progress further into a pose, test it first, but remember that form, alignment, breathing and stability take priority. Listen to your body. If you feel pain or discomfort, that's more than a gentle stretch. Don't force the movement. If you are working for progression, test the transition shortly before you return to the start position.

If you're struggling with a specific movement, e.g., due to limited balance, strength, or range of motion and want to improve, you could consider contacting a local yoga instructor who can help identify and address the underlying issues.

The poses

In this guide, each pose has been broken down into levels to make them achievable for beginners and to give options for further development. The progression levels for each pose are set out to be used as a step-by-step process, building on the step before challenging balance, stability, strength and flexibility in slightly larger increments than the previous.

The first level (level 1) will be a continuation from one of the starting positions detailed earlier in the guide, so before attempting level 1 for any yoga pose from this section, it is advised that you are comfortable with, understand, and can hold the appropriate starting position.

As you progress through the levels of each pose, you should always practice the principals of the previous as per the description, even if you are simply moving through that level to get to the next. This will keep you focused, mindful and aligned, resulting in a more effective session.

If you find that you are unable to progress to the next level for certain exercises as it's uncomfortable, range of movement is limited, or balance is an issue, you have found your progression point. Hold here for a few sessions and then test the next progression again.

For greater understanding, there is a breakdown of each pose with muscle groups worked, along with a ranking system of relevance for strength, stability, flexibility and balance. The system uses 1-5, with 5 being the most relevant and 1 being the least relevant. This may be useful if you are looking to tailor your workouts towards a stronger focus on one of the five pillars mentioned earlier. Also in the overview of each pose, there is a QR code or link that can be scanned for an animated version of the exercise that combines all levels mentioned. This may be useful for further clarity.

Tree Pose

Starting position: Standing

Balance: 5

The "go to" pose for balance development. Focused coordination is needed to maintain a single-leg stance, especially without support options.

Stability: 4

Engages core and leg muscles significantly to keep the body upright and aligned, especially during longer holds.

Strength: 3

Builds strength in the standing leg and core.

Flexibility: 2

Requires mild hip opening to position the foot on the inner thigh or calf.

Muscle Groups Used:

Quadriceps (upper front of leg), glutes (buttocks and hip area), core (abs, lower back, and other stabilising muscles), ankle stabilisers, calfs.

Extra information: Tree Pose is a standing balance pose that strengthens the muscles of the legs and core while developing stability. It gently opens the hip of the lifted leg to add an element of flexibility in this area.

Once you have performed the pose on one leg in your workout, mirror the exercise on the other side. When you reach the maximum level, try this with your eyes closed for an extra challenge.

Level 1

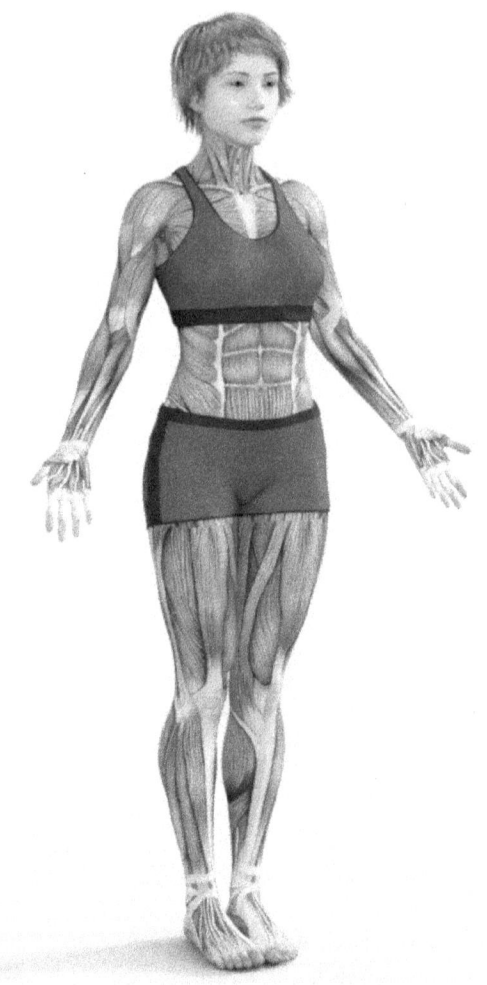

- From the standing start position, place your feet together and firmly on the ground with an even weight distribution throughout
- Bend your knees slightly so they are not locked
- Keep your core engaged and your head in a neutral position
- Arms by your sides and lifted slightly away from your body, palms facing forward

Level 2

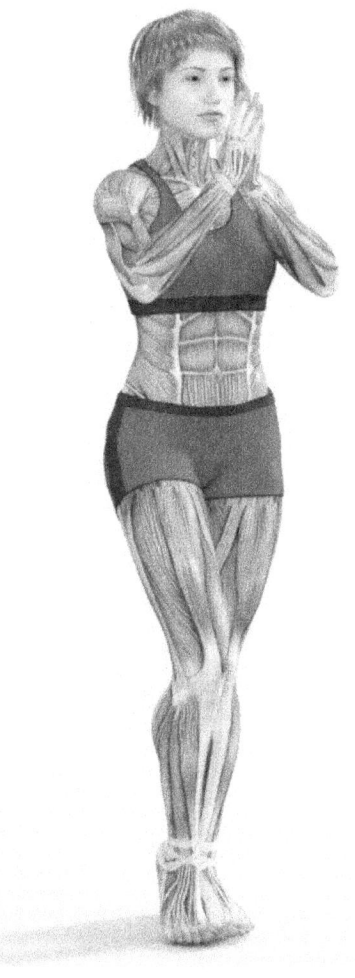

- Slowly shift most of your bodyweight to your left foot and lift the heel of your right foot away from the floor. Maintain hip alignment while you do this
- Lift and bend your arms to place your palms together in front of your face
- Ensure you keep your shoulders back and down to maintain spinal alignment

Level 3

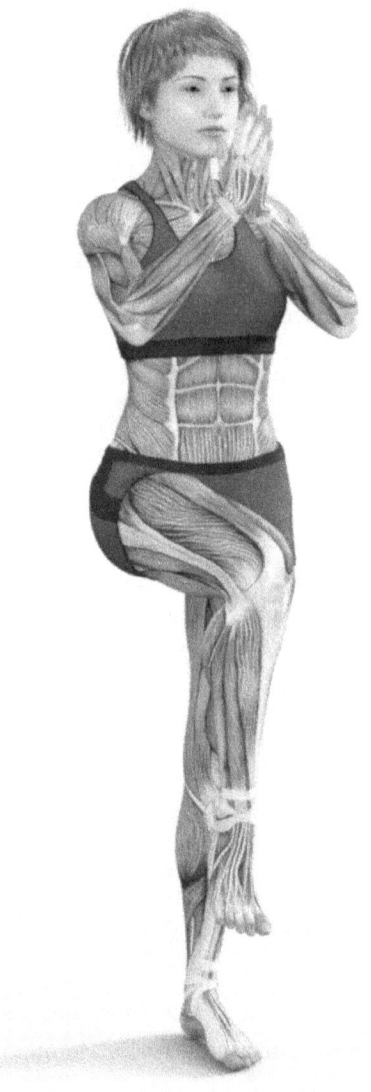

- Slowly shift the remainder of your body weight to your left foot while maintaining alignment in your hips
- Maintaining the slight bend in your left leg, lift your right leg and bend at the knee to create a right angle between your hamstring and calf

Level 4

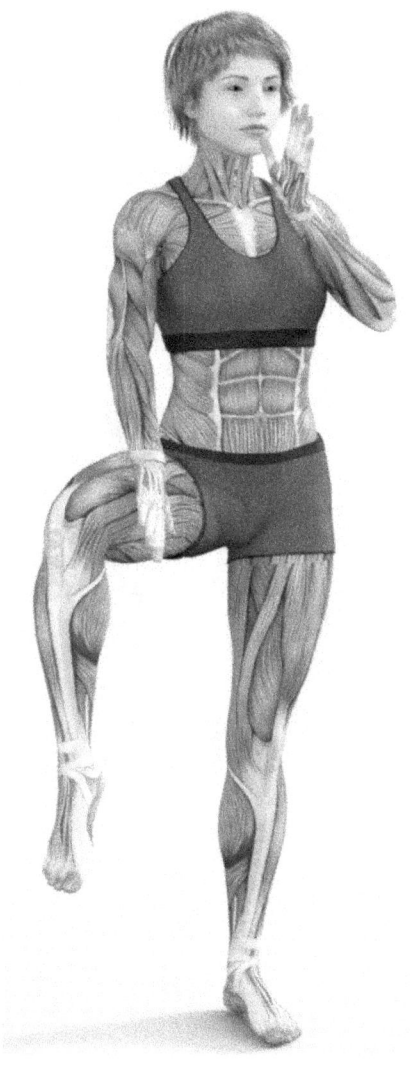

- Keep your left hand in position and lower your so your palm connects with the inside of your right leg
- Extend your right hip backwards, applying gentle pressure through your palm if necessary
- Maintain the elevation of your right leg and alignment of your hips as you do this

Level 5

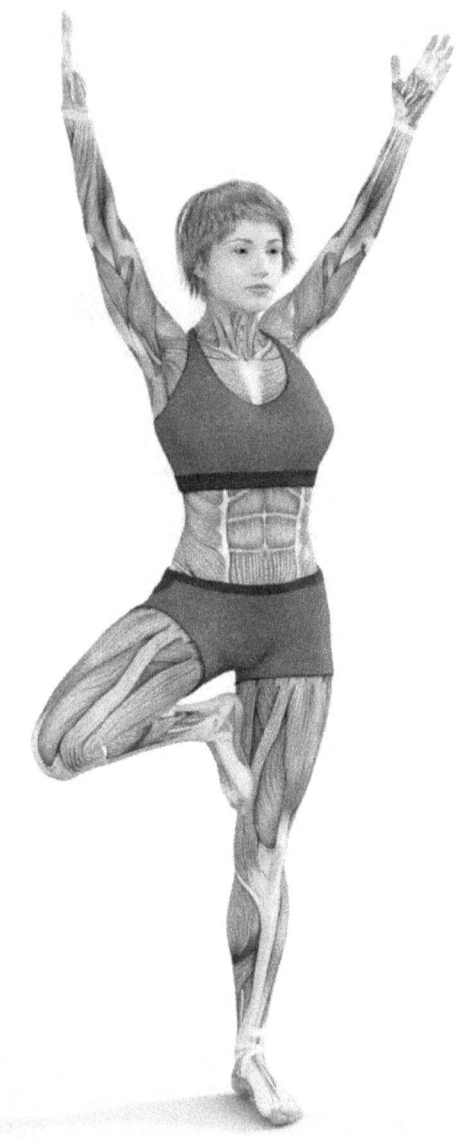

- Maintain the extension of your right leg and bend at the knee to bring the sole of your foot flat against your inner left leg
- Maintaining your alignment, raise your arms above your head. Palms can be flat together or facing inwards at a bigger angle

Support option

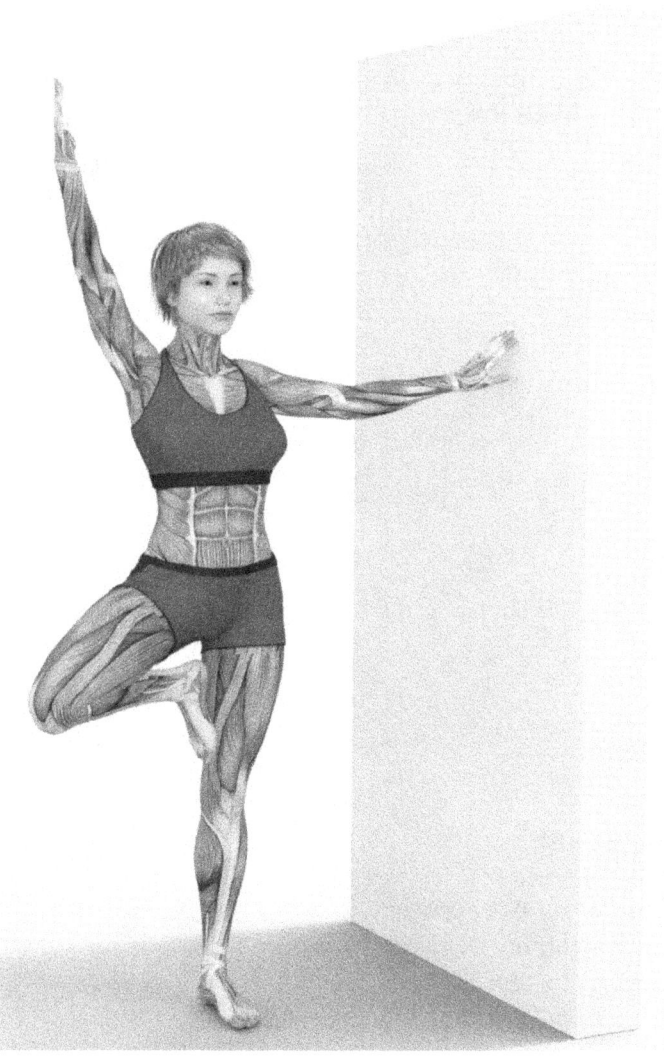

- A solid wall or sturdy chair can be used for support
- If you choose to use a support, use minimal contact, fingertips or a light palm placement

Warrior

Scan for animation

Starting position: <u>Standing</u>

Strength: <u>5</u>

A strong lunge pose to engage multiple muscle groups throughout the body, including legs, glutes, core, and upper body.

Stability: <u>4</u>

Demands significant core and lower body stability to keep the torso aligned, especially with your arms raised.

Flexibility: <u>3</u>

Chest opening, a gentle stretch in the back leg's hip flexors and hamstrings.

Balance: <u>2</u>

Balance is challenged slightly to maintain the pose, but the wide stance provides more stability than some other poses.

Muscle Groups Used:

Quadriceps and hamstrings (front and back upper leg), glutes (buttocks), core (abs, lower back, and other stabiliser muscles), deltoids and trapezius (shoulders and upper back), adductors (inner thighs), calfs (rear, lower legs).

Extra information: Warrior pose is a powerful standing pose that builds strength in the legs, glutes, core, and upper body. Stability is developed in the lunge and engaged core, with flexibility development in the hips and chest. There is a small challenge to balance.

Once you have completed the warrior pose, repeat so the opposite leg is forward facing.

Level 1

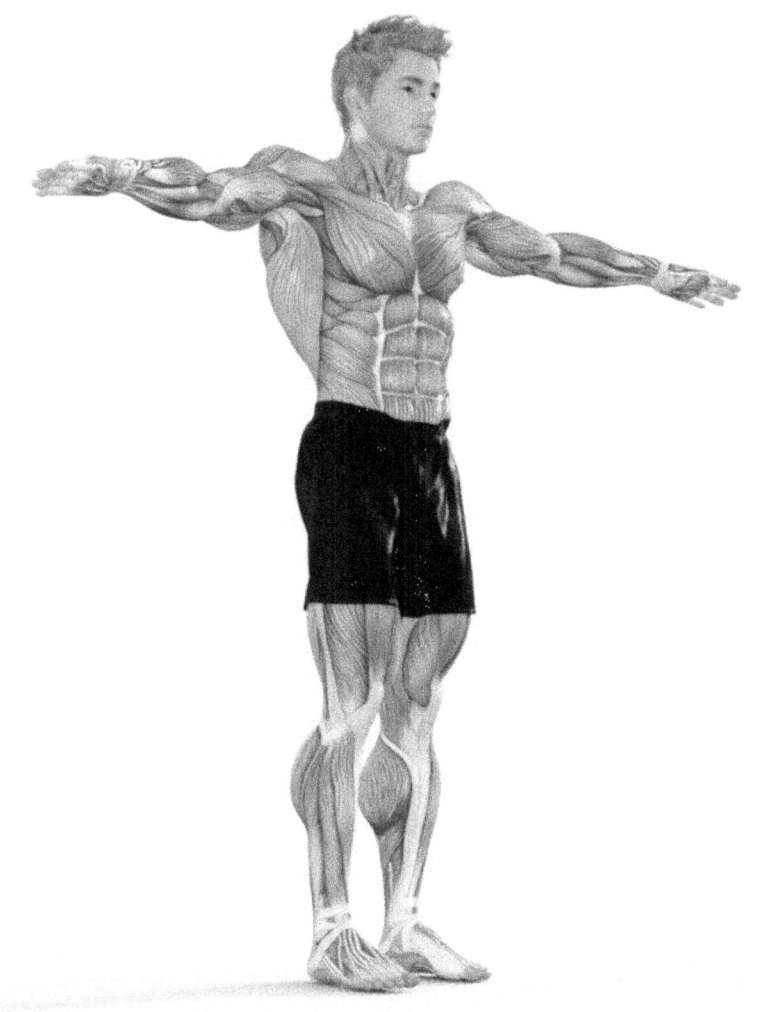

- From the standing start position, plant your feet firmly on the floor about hip width apart
- Raise your arms out to your sides until they are parallel with the ground, palms facing down
- Head in a neutral position, maintain core engagement and alignment

Level 2

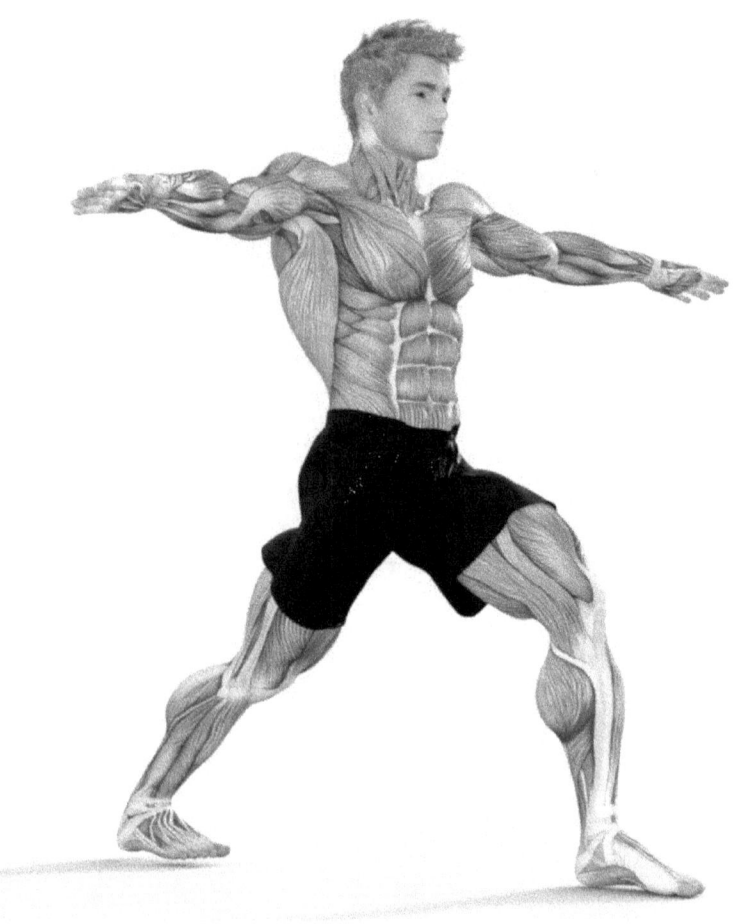

- Step forward with your left leg, bending at the knee. The knee should be directly above the ankle
- Distribute your body weight evenly through the soles of your feet
- Keep your arms raised for balance

Level 3

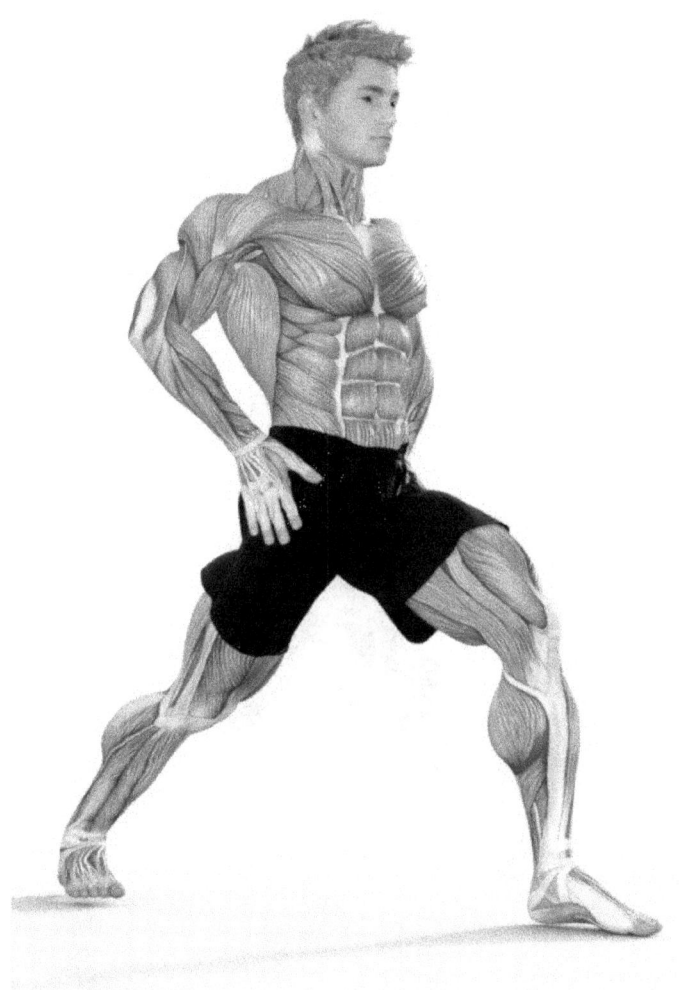

- Slowly re position the foot of your rear leg so your toes point at a forty-five degree angle from your midline and redistribute most of your bodyweight on this foot to the outside edge
- Lower your arms to place your palms on your hips

Level 4

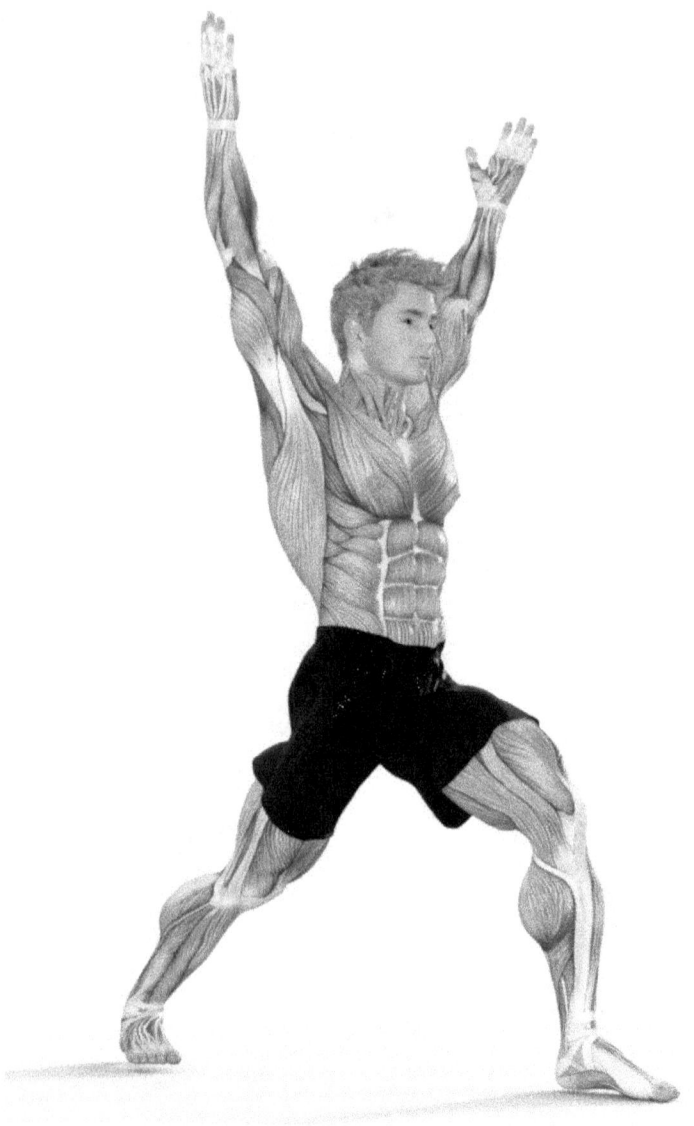

- Keeping your feet firmly planted on the ground, straighten your arms and raise them above your head, palms facing inwards
- Hips should maintain alignment throughout, be aware of hip tilt

Eagle

Starting position: <u>Standing</u>

Balance: <u>5</u>

The single-leg stance with crossed legs and crossed arms challenges balance significantly.

Flexibility: <u>4</u>

Develops flexibility to a high level in several parts of the body. Upper and lower.

Stability: <u>4</u>

The single-leg position challenges stability and focus fairly intensely.

Strength: <u>3</u>

Develops a degree of strength in the legs and core, but not as intensely as some other poses.

Muscle Groups Used:

Quadriceps (leg), glutes (buttocks), core (abs lower back and other stabiliser muscles), hip abductors/adductors (inner and outer upper leg), rhomboids and trapezius (upper back), deltoids (shoulders), hamstrings (upper, rear leg), ankle stabilisers, wrist flexors/extensors (for arms).

Extra information: Eagle Pose is a single-leg exercise designed to challenge balance and flexibility in the hips, shoulders, upper back and forearms. The higher levels of eagle can feel uncomfortable and restrictive for many due to the "wrapped, compressed" posture, so working up to it may take longer than other poses. Take your time.

Level 1

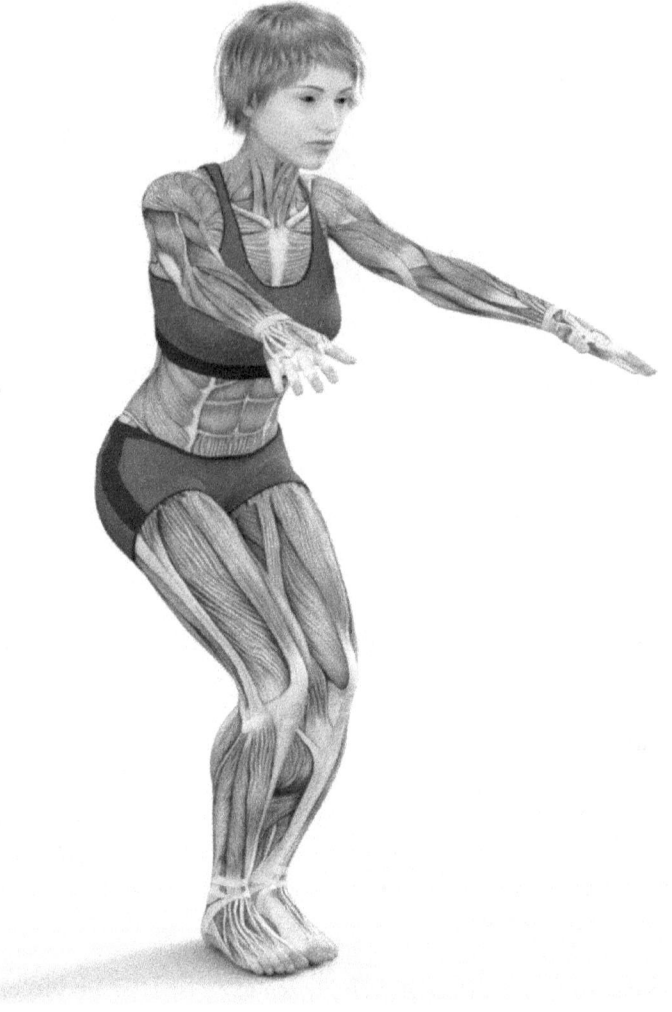

- From the standing start position, bring your feet and knees together with your body weight evenly distributed through your soles
- Lift your arms to your front for balance
- Maintain alignment and core engagement as you bend at the knees to enter the start of a sitting movement

Level 2

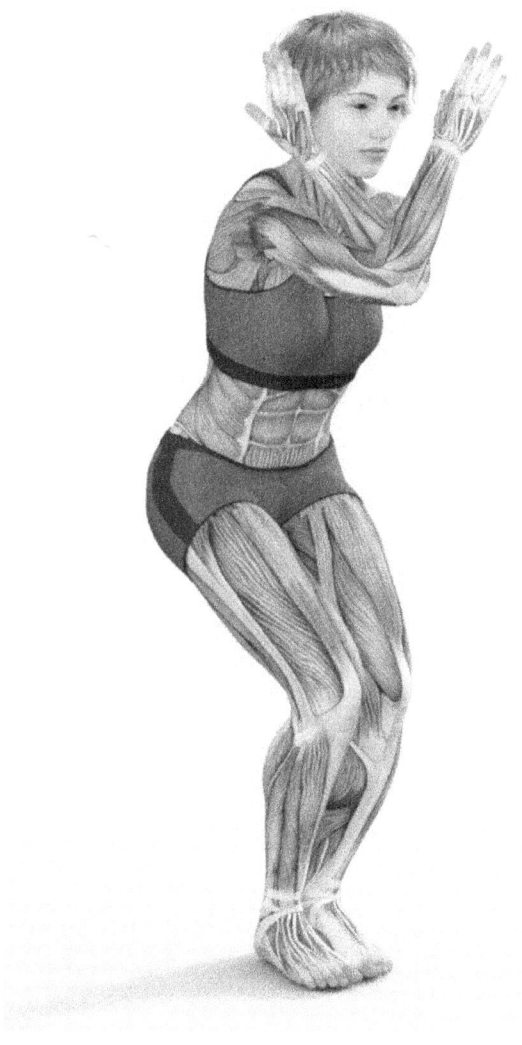

- Maintain your lower body position and even weight distribution through your feet
- Move your arms up and across your body, bending at the elbows to form a "V" shape with your upper arms in front of your face
- Palms facing out to your sides

Level 3

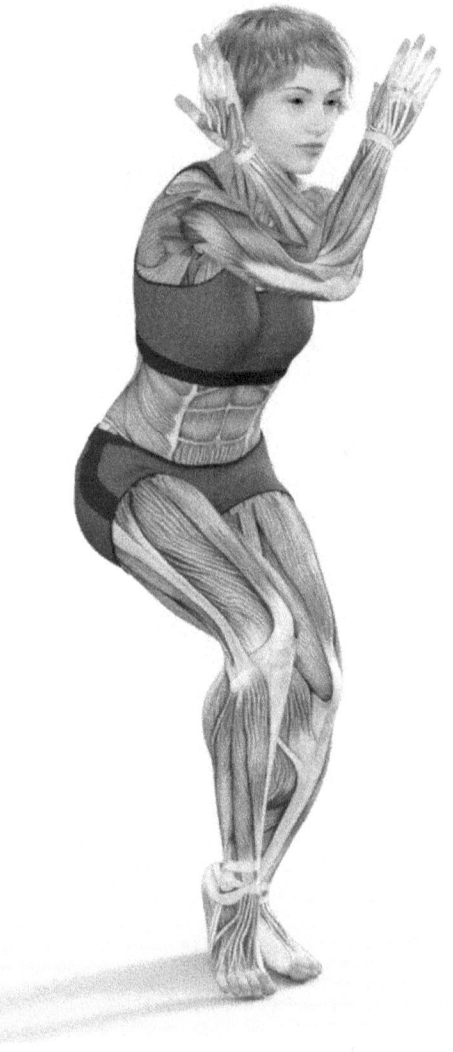

- Maintain hip alignment and core engagement as you shift the majority of your body weight to your left foot
- Bend the knee of your right foot to lift the heel off the ground
- Maintain upper body position

Level 4

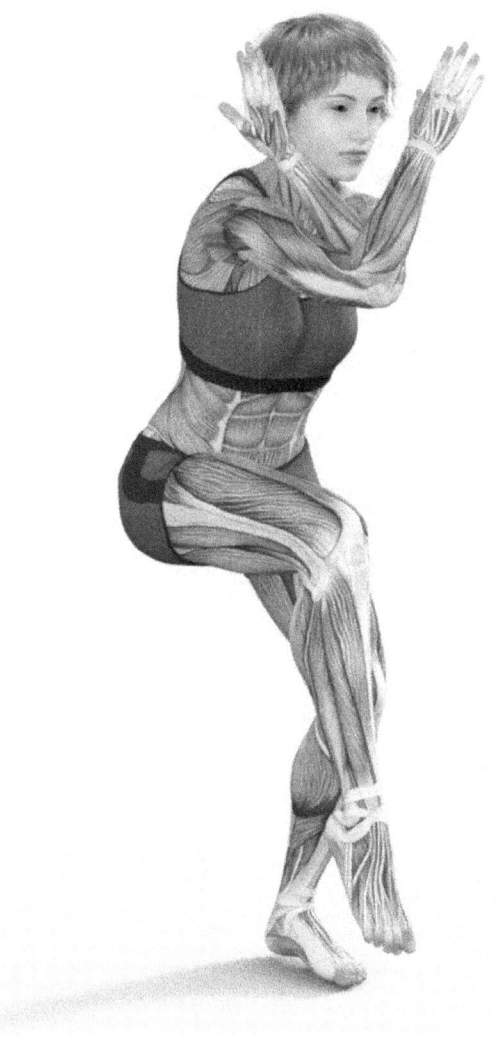

- Lift your right leg so your upper leg is parallel with the ground
- Bend your knee and point your toes
- Be aware of possible hip tilt, loss of core engagement and general alignment practice at this point

Level 5

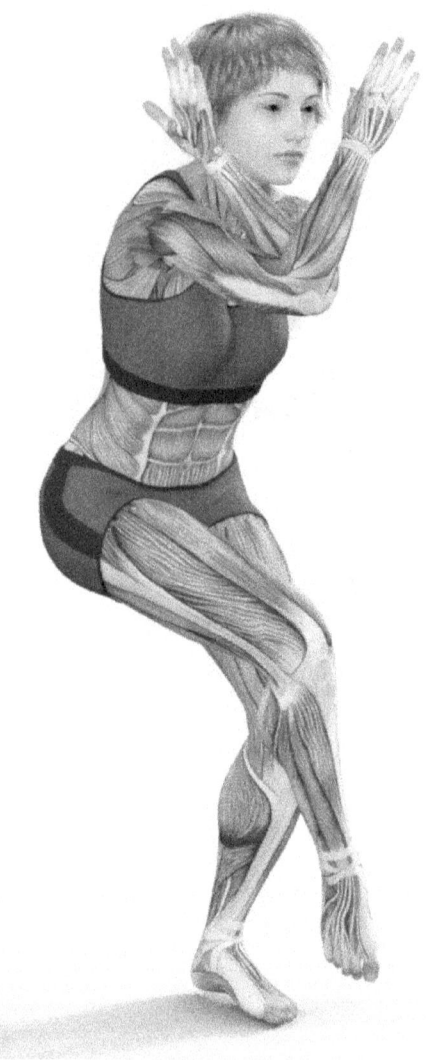

- Slowly move your right leg across the front of your body to place your calf muscle on the knee of your left leg
- Keep the toes of your right leg pointed and ensure your left foot stays planted evenly on the ground

Level 6

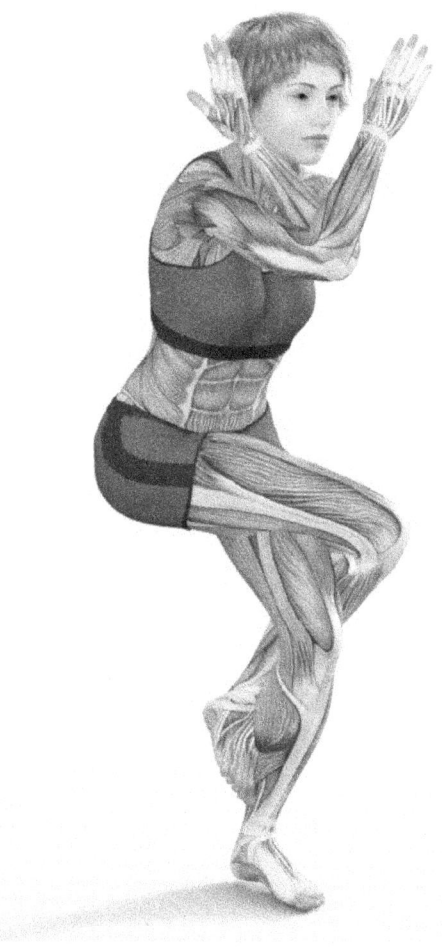

- Continue the right leg movement further by lifting higher and twisting through the quadriceps and wrap your upper right foot around your left calf muscle
- Maintain alignment, core engagement and even weight distribution through your planted foot and be aware of unwanted hip tilt through all levels

Dancer

Scan for animation

Start position: standing

Balance: 5

The single-leg stance, forward hip hinge and raised leg challenge balance and focus at an advanced level.

Flexibility: 5

Higher levels of this pose develop flexibility in multiple areas of the body to a high level.

Strength: 4

Builds considerable strength in the lower body and core.

Stability: 4

Stability is also challenged significantly when maintaining this pose.

Muscle Groups Used:

Quadriceps, glutes, core, hip flexors, hamstrings, deltoids and trapezius, rhomboids, ankle stabilisers, latissimus dorsi, wrist flexors/extensors.

Extra information: Dancer pose is an excellent standing exercise that challenges strength, balance, flexibility and stability, to around the same degree. The higher levels of dancer pose in this guide are considered advanced. If you find balance is causing a delay in progression, you can choose to use a support, such as a wall or sturdy chair, to steady yourself. You should make light contact with your hand or fingertips rather than use this support as a crutch.

Once you have completed the dancer to your chosen level, repeat with the opposite leg raised.

Level 1

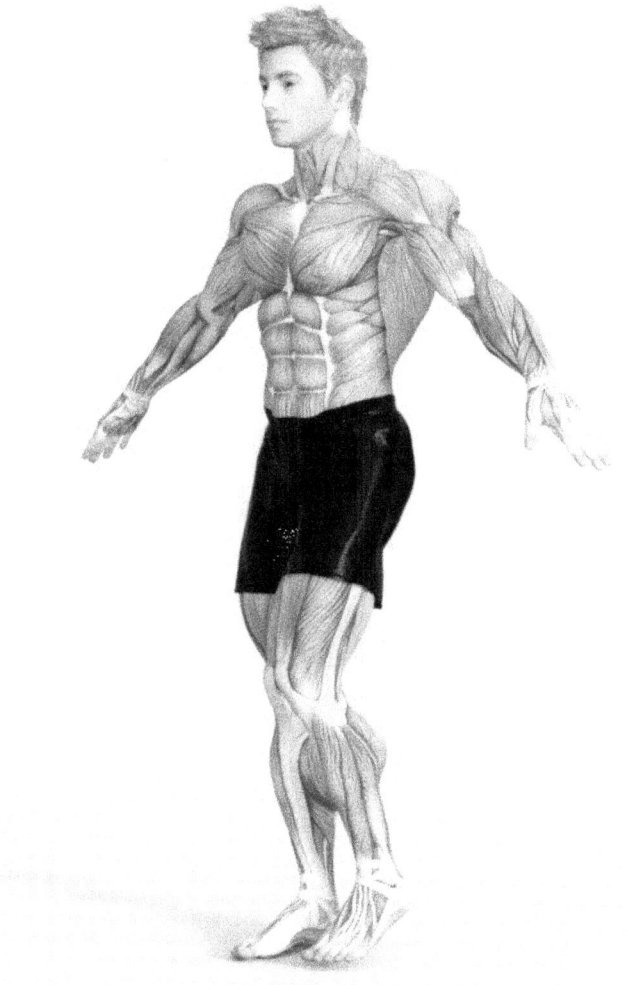

- From the standing start position, ensure your weight is distributed evenly through the sole of your right foot
- Raise your arms to your sides slightly for balance
- Lift your left foot up and away from the ground by bending your left knee and moving your upper leg upwards
- Your toes of your left foot should be just clear of the floor

Level 2

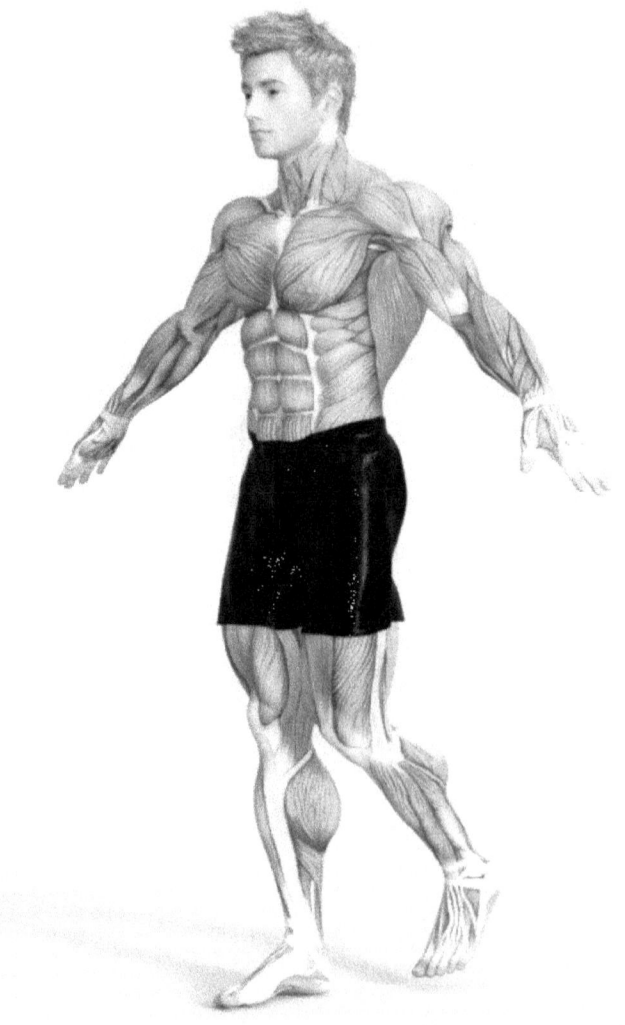

- Slowly increase the bend in your left knee and align your upper left leg with your right
- Maintaining the bend in your left knee will place your lower left leg behind you
- Your left foot should not make contact with the floor

Level 3

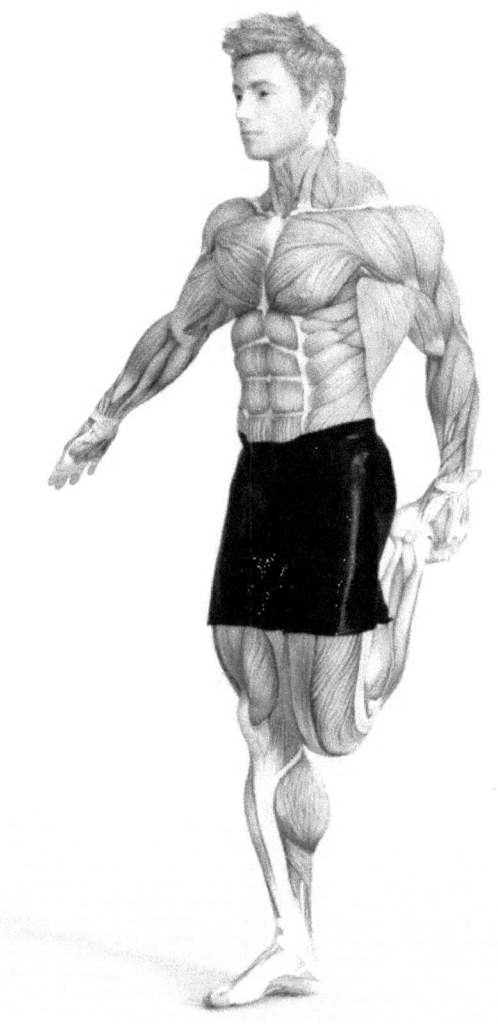

- Maintain alignment, core engagement and be aware of hip tilt as you bend your left leg at the knee
- Grasp your left foot with your left hand and pull your knee towards your midline. Both knees should make contact
- Be aware of unwanted forward hip tilt at this point

Level 4

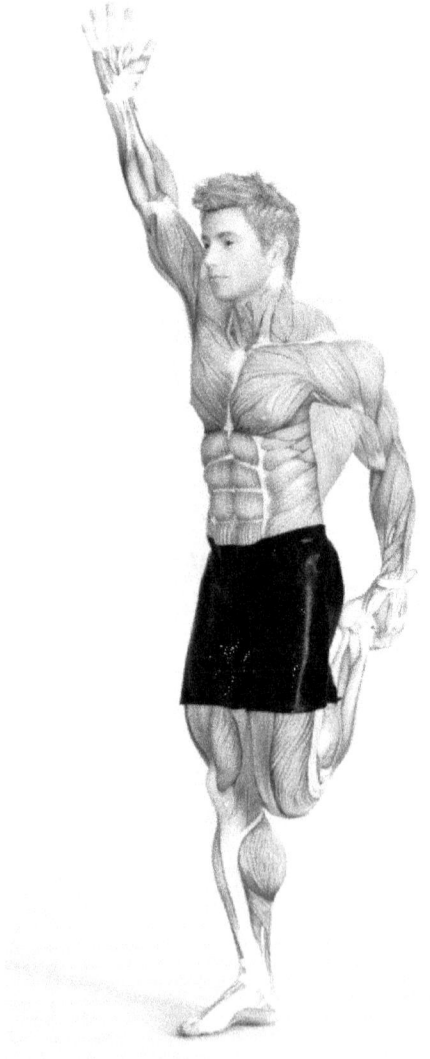

- Maintain alignment throughout. Ensure your planted foot is evenly loaded with your body weight
- Once you are stable in this position, raise your right arm, straight, out to your side, and above your head, palm facing inwards

Level 5

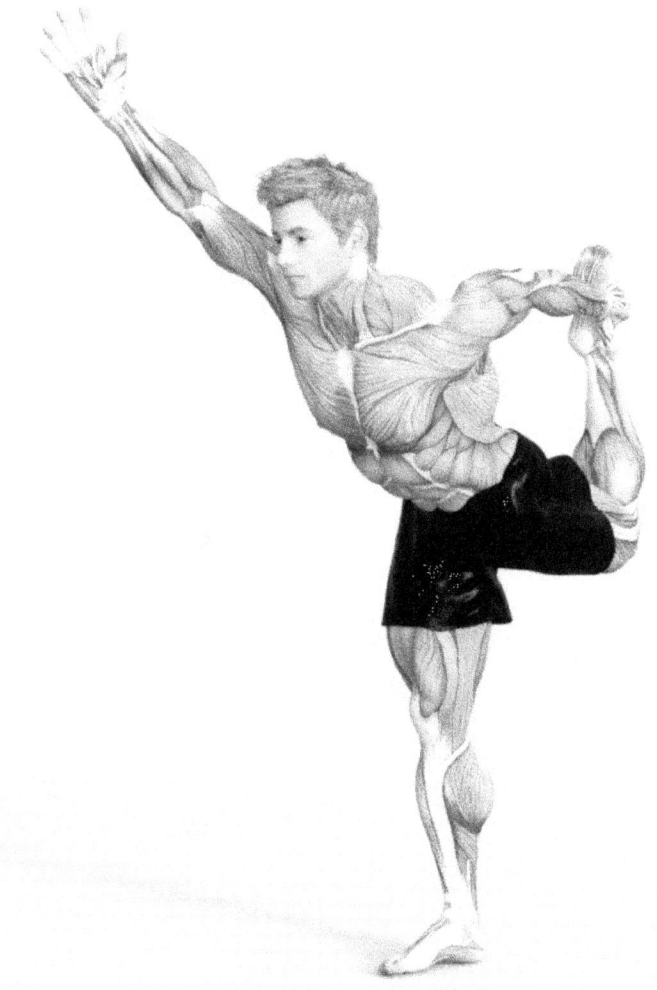

- Maintain alignment, core engagement, and be aware of unwanted hip tilt (to your right) as you hinge forward at the hips
- During this movement, your left leg will naturally move up and backwards. Increase this movement when you are comfortable for further range of movement
- Ensure the knee of your planted foot does not lock throughout the pose

Support option

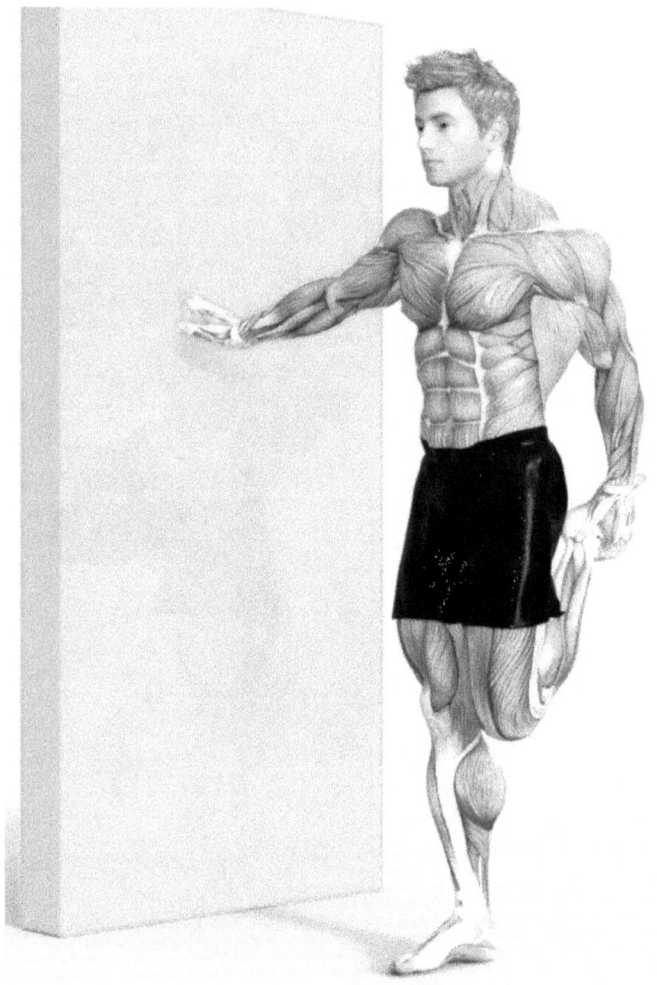

- Options for support can be used in the earlier stages of this pose
- I'd suggest using support up to level 3 of this pose, as we should be confident and developed in the balancing element of this pose before progressing to further levels

Chair

Starting position: Standing

Strength: 5

The squatting movement is a strong position that develops strength in the legs core and back.

Scan for animation

Stability: 4

Stability in the core and lower body is challenged significantly, especially with arms raised.

Balance: 3

Balance is challenged moderately to maintain the position, but this pose starts with a strong base with both feet on the ground.

Flexibility: 2

Flexibility is not the main focus of this pose. There is, however, a gentle challenge in this area when arms are raised.

Muscle Groups Used: Quadriceps, glutes, core, erector spinae, deltoids and trapezius, hamstrings, adductors, rhomboids, soleus and gastrocnemius.

Extra information: Chair pose is a powerful standing pose that builds strength in the legs, glutes, and core while developing stability with the low squat. An element of balance is needed to maintain alignment. A gentle stretch in the shoulders and upper back is the limit of flexibility. Performing a deeper squat will add more intensity and challenge to this pose.

Level 1

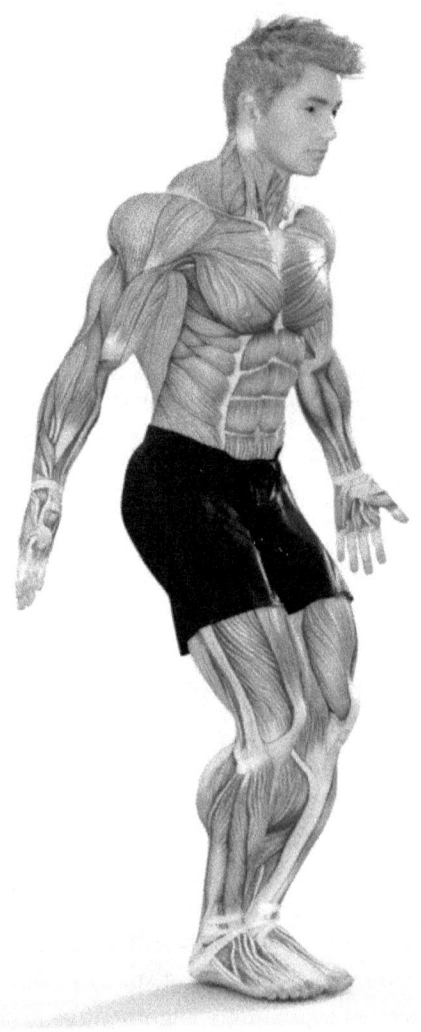

- From the standing start position, bring your feet and knees together, toes pointing forward. Ensure your weight is evenly distributed through the soles of both feet
- Bend your knees slightly to place you into a shallow squat
- Lift your arms out to your sides slightly for balance

Level 2

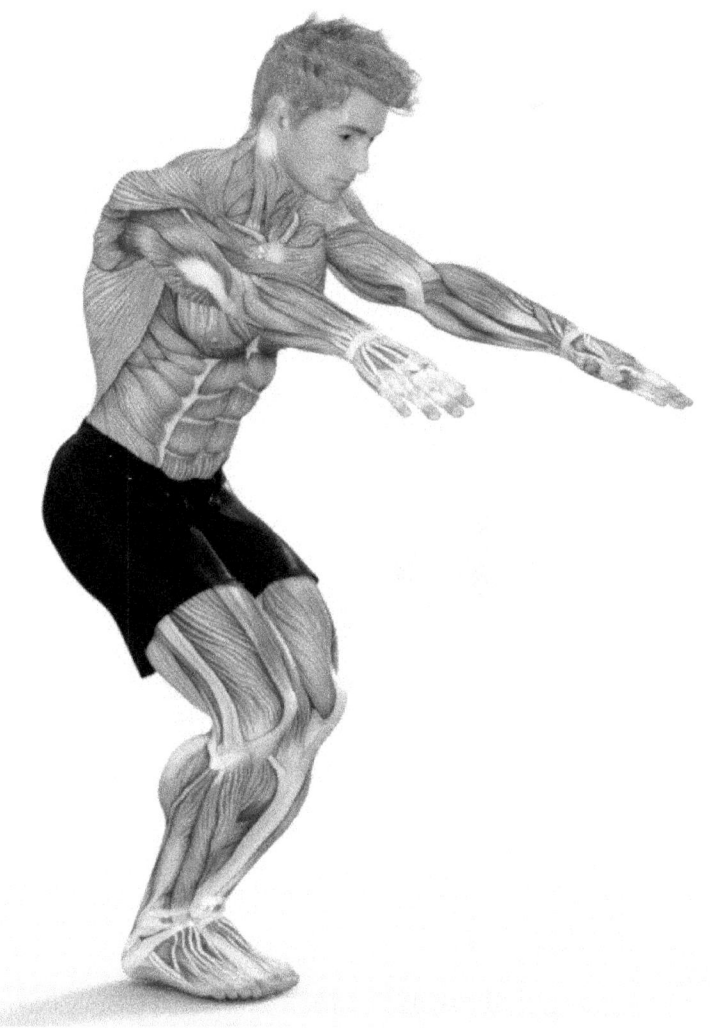

- Raise your arms straight and to your front, palms down for balance
- Slowly sit down into a deeper squat
- Be aware of your back and hip alignment to ensure you don't hinge forward through your hips
- Maintain even weight distribution through your feet

Level 3

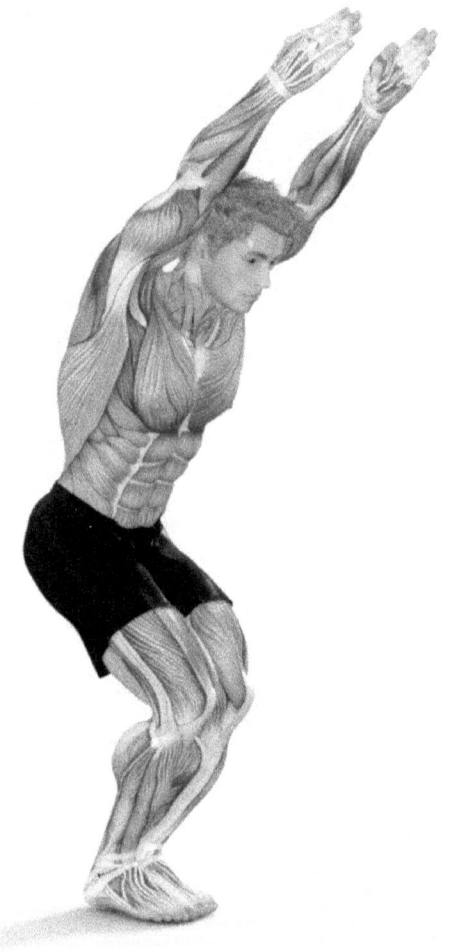

- While maintaining the shallow squat position and paying attention to alignment, core engagement, raise your straight arms up and above your head, palms facing inwards
- Arms should be a continuation of your back alignment
- Keep your head in a neutral position for balance and to help maintain alignment

Level 4

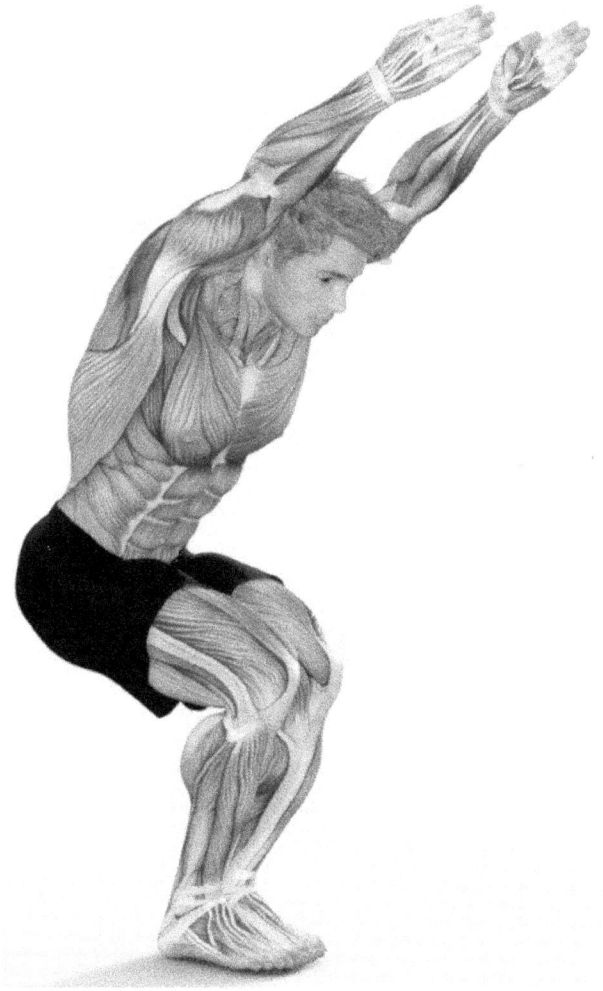

- Slowly sit deeper into the squatting movement until you form a ninety-degree angle between your upper and lower rear legs
- Even weight distribution through the feet, core engagement and correct alignment should be maintained throughout this pose
- If shoulder mobility allows, the hands can be clasped together above the head

Support option

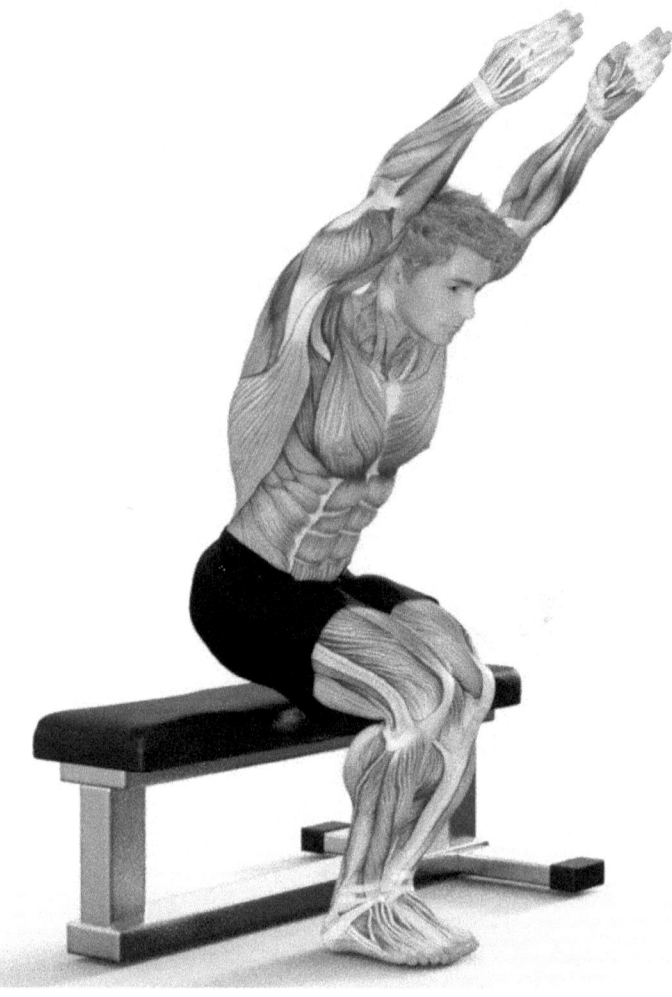

- A support option for this pose can be a sturdy chair or workout bench
- Place this behind you and view it as an "insurance policy" in case you lose your balance
- A workout bench or low chair could also be used as a measure; Once your glutes are about to make contact, you will be close, or hit the ninety-degree angle of the rear leg bend

Four-Limbed Staff Pose

Start position: Four point

Strength: 5

This pose engages the upper body and core intensely, developing strength throughout.

Scan for animation

Stability: 5

Stability and strength are equally challenged in this pose, as maintaining alignment and supporting the body's weight can be equally demanding.

Balance: 3

There is a small amount of balance development involved to maintain alignment, but it is a four point contact pose giving a fairly stable base.

Flexibility: 1

Minimal flexibility is involved as the main focus is on strength and stability.

Muscle Groups Used:

Pectoralis major (chest), triceps (rear, upper arms), deltoids (shoulders), core (abdominals, lower back and other stabilisers), serratus anterior (side of chest), quadriceps (upper front leg), gluteus maximus (buttocks), rhomboids (rear shoulder).

Extra information: Four-Limbed staff pose is an intense pose to develop strength in the chest, arms, shoulders, and core, but is also excellent for the development of stability throughout. When starting out, be aware of dropping the stomach to the floor or raising the hips. This can creep up, so it may be useful to glance sidelong into a mirror during the pose.

Level 1

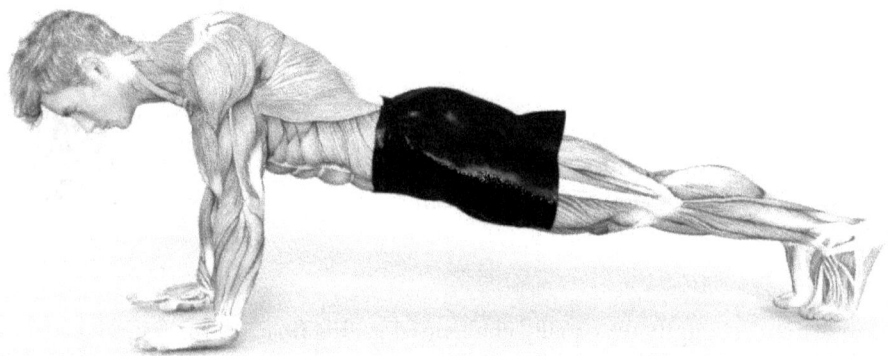

- From the four point start position, straighten your legs to transfer your lower body weight through your toes instead of your knees. Feet should be about hip width apart
- Engage your core and maintain alignment, ensuring your abdominals and hips do not sink towards the ground or lift towards the sky
- Palms should be flat to the floor underneath the shoulders and spaced about shoulder width apart

Level 2

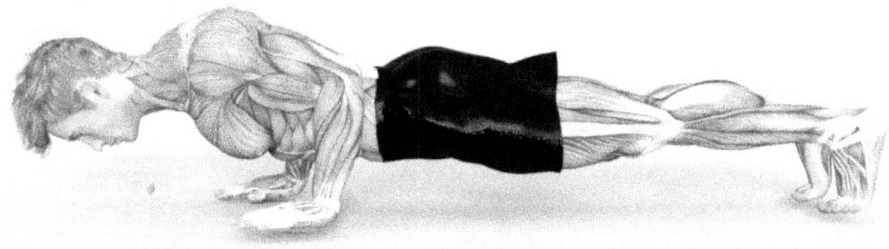

- Maintain alignment and core engagement as you slowly lower your upper body towards the ground by bending at the elbows
- During this movement, ensure your elbows do not flare out to your sides
- Lower until your body is parallel with the ground
- Core engagement and alignment should be monitored throughout the pose

Bridge pose

Start position: Supine

Strength: 4

Strong engagement of the core and back muscles for good strength development in these areas.

Flexibility: 4

Good stretching opportunities in the hips and upper body for flexibility development.

Stability: 3

Core and lower body engagement to maintain alignment in the lift.

Balance: 1

Minimal balance challenge as the pose is performed lying down with feet, shoulders and arms planted.

Muscle Groups Used:

Gluteus maximus (buttocks), hamstrings (upper, rear legs), core (abdominals, lower back and other stabilisers), erector spinae (deep back muscle), quadriceps (upper front leg), pectoralis major (chest), anterior deltoids (front shoulder), rhomboids and trapezius (rear shoulder).

Extra information: Bridge pose is a beginner "backbend" used to strengthen the glutes, hamstrings, and core. Some find this uncomfortable on the neck or back of the head due to pressure from the floor. A small pillow, foam pad can be placed behind the head, or rolled-up towel under the neck to alleviate this.

Level 1

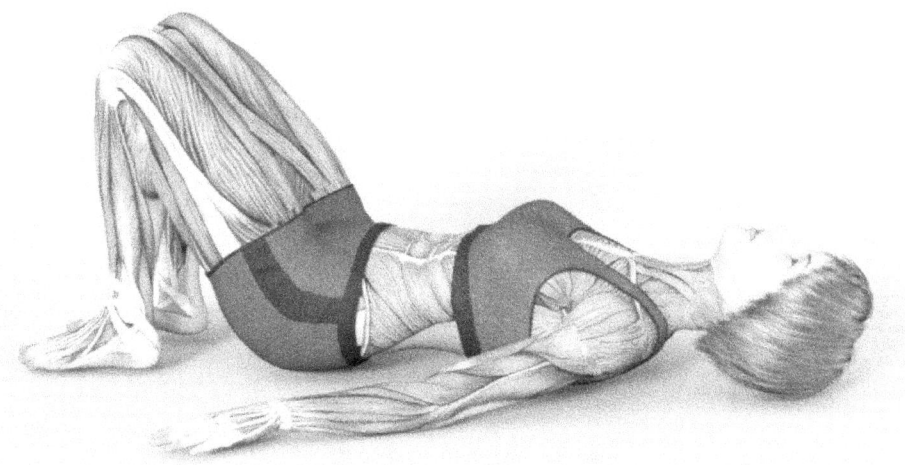

- From the supine starting position, bring your feet and knees together so your feet are about hip width apart
- Position your feet so your ankles are stacked underneath your knees, toes pointing forward
- Apply pressure evenly through your feet and backs of your shoulders

<u>Level 2</u>

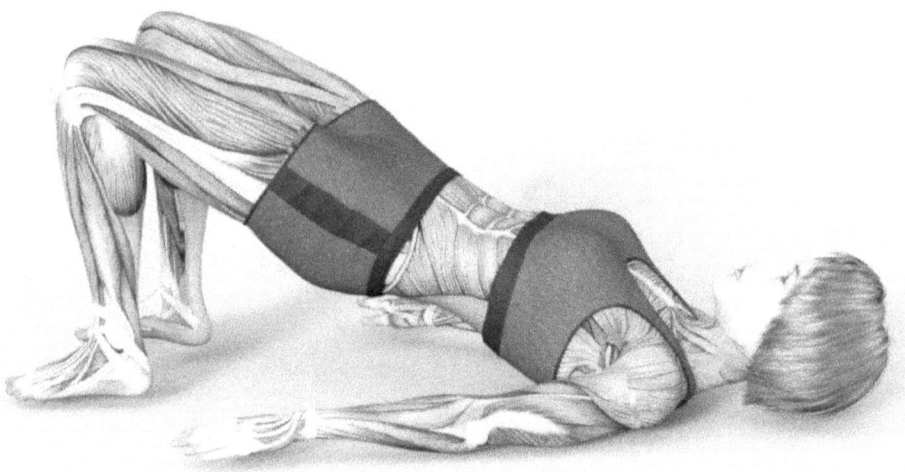

- Maintaining core engagement, push through your feet to bring your hips upwards
- Continue the movement until you reach alignment with your chest, abdominals and upper front legs
- Knees should not flare outwards or inwards
- Support can be used behind the neck if this is uncomfortable. A small pillow or rolled-up towel are common options for support

Forward fold

Start position: Seated on floor

Flexibility: 5

Scan for animation

Intense stretch for the hamstrings, even during the start position for some, extending to other parts of the body as the levels increase.

Strength: 3

Moderate core engagement involved to maintain alignment and support in the forward bend.

Stability: 3

Moderate core and leg engagement to stabilise the body in the folded position.

Balance: 2

Gentle balance development to keep alignment, but there is a lot of contact with the ground during this pose to provide stability.

Muscle Groups Used:

Hamstrings (upper rear legs), Calves (lower rear leg), erector spinae (lower back), core (abdominals, lower back and other stabilisers), gluteus maximus (buttocks), quadriceps (upper front legs), latissimus dorsi (back).

Other information: Forward fold can be an intense flexibility development pose from the starting position as the hamstrings are immediately challenged. As the range of movement increases, more muscle groups are incorporated. Small increments of forward movement can be used to increase the challenge, especially for those with tight hamstrings.

Level 1

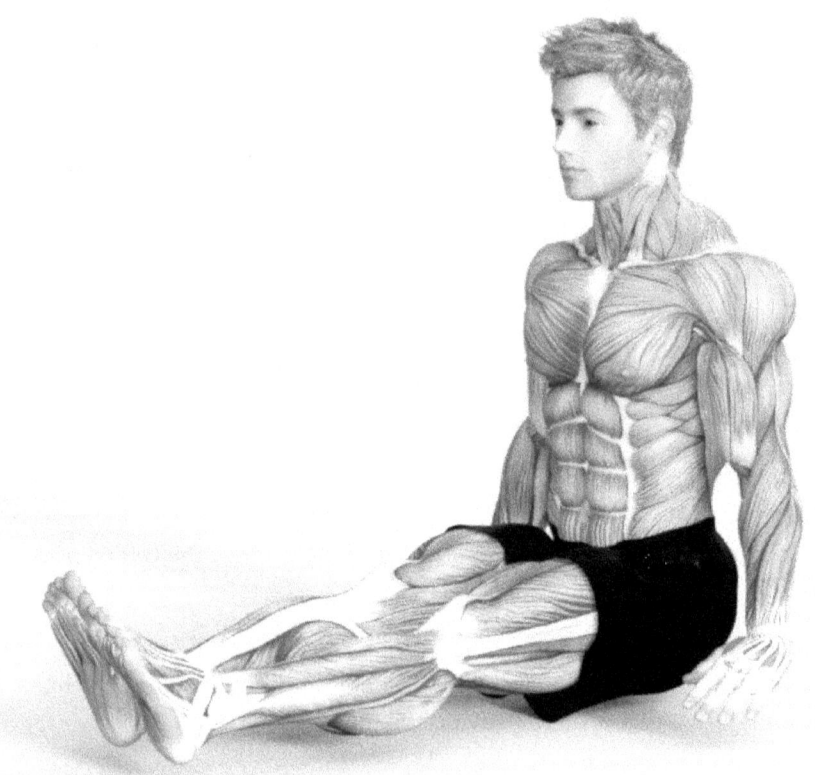

- From the seated on floor position, move your upper body forward slightly to sit with a flat back
- Arms by your sides, making gentle contact with the ground
- Straighten your legs and position your feet and knees about hip width apart, toes pointing forward

Level 2

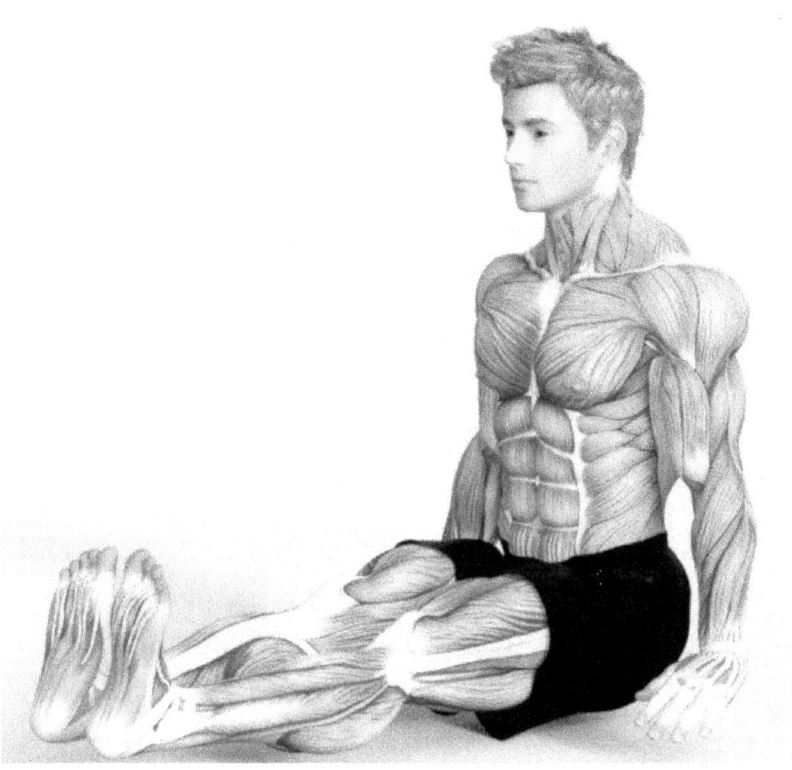

- While maintaining core engagement, slowly pull your toes towards your body by hinging at the ankles
- This should engage your hamstrings

Level 3

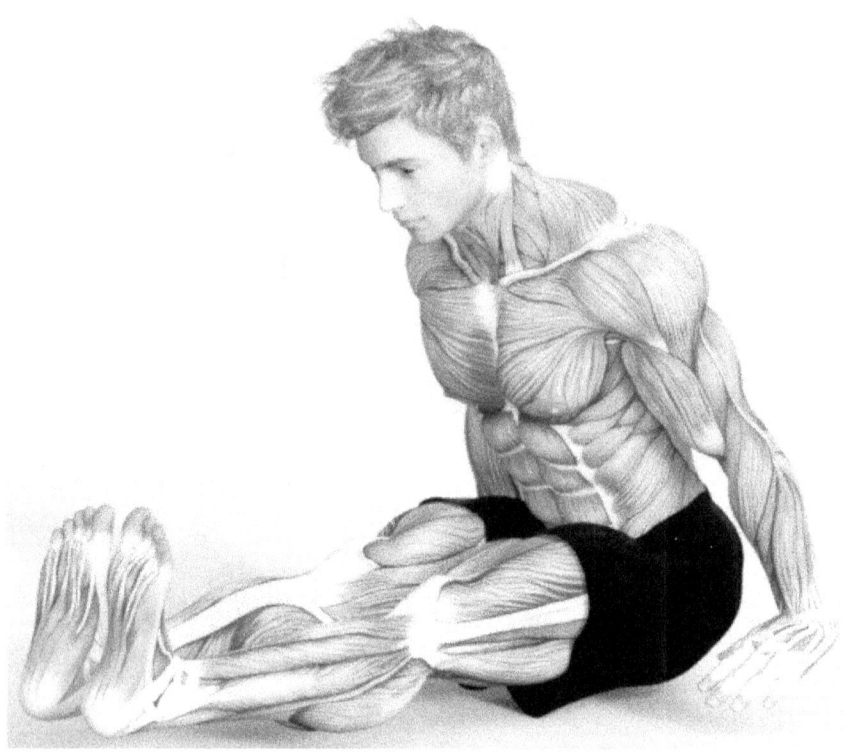

- Keeping your toes pointed, hinge at the hips to move your upper body towards your legs
- This can be intense with small incremental movements, so must be performed slowly

Level 4

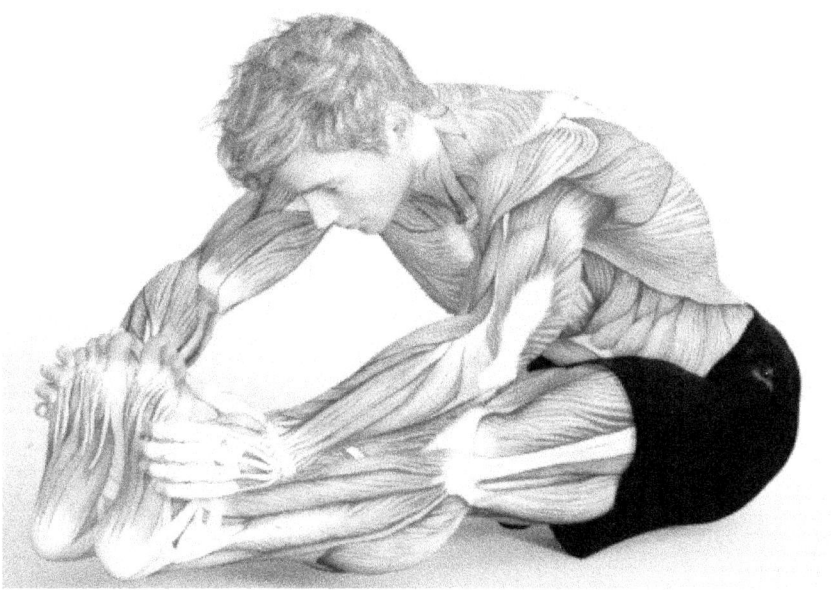

- While maintaining the ankle bend (toes pointed) continue the forward fold movement by increasing the forward hip hinge
- Slight forward flexion of the upper spine at this point can be used to enhance spinal flexibility
- If pain free flexibility allows, reach forward with your hands to grasp your feet

Level 5

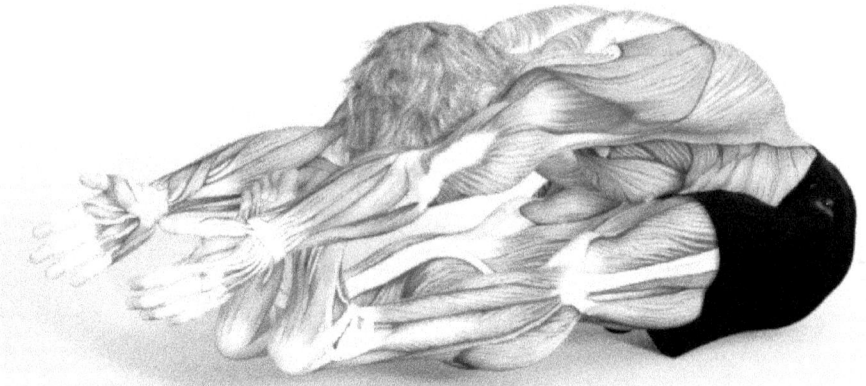

- Maintain core engagement as you increase the forward fold further
- Slight flexion of the upper spine can be used to add flexibility to the spine at this point also
- Reach forward with your hands, arms straight to challenge strength while in this pose

Cobra

Start position: Prone

Flexibility: 4

This pose challenges flexibility through the spine, chest and abdominals fairly significantly, depending on the level worked at.

Strength: 4

Scan for animation

Strength is also a key player in this pose, as in higher levels of this pose, muscle groups are required to lift and hold body weight.

Stability: 3

Your core and legs engage just enough to keep your pelvis grounded for stability.

Balance: 2

Balance isn't a big deal here, as you have a large contact area. Mindfulness is, however, still needed to maintain alignment.

Muscle Groups Used:

Erector spinae (long muscles along your spine), latissimus dorsi (mid-back), trapezius and rhomboids (upper back), core (abs and obliques), gluteus maximus (your butt), quadriceps (front thighs), pectoralis major (chest), deltoids (shoulders).

Other Information:

Cobra pose can be an intense backbend movement, especially for those who are not used to movement on this plane. It's great for opening up the chest and giving the spine some extension. If you are new to this pose, a small amount of movement can be excellent for tension release. Start at lower levels with slow and steady movement. Look for improved range of motion in the spine before progressing to the removal of support from your hands.

Level 1

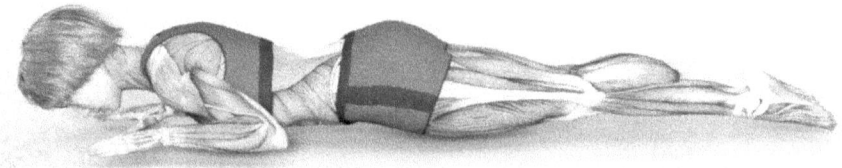

- From the prone start position, apply even pressure through your palms, hips and fronts of your upper legs
- Legs straight and head in a neutral position
- Maintain alignment through your spine and core engagement

Level 2

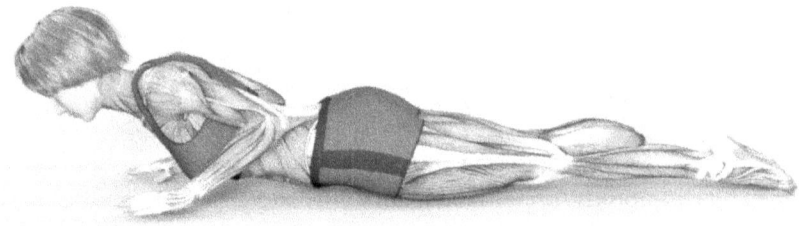

- Position your palms so they are in line with your chest and about shoulder with apart
- Push through your palms to slightly extend your lower back

Level 3

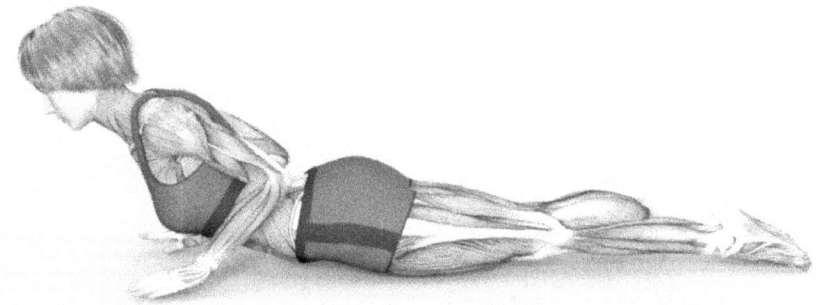

- Slowly continue the back extension by applying more pressure through the palms
- Maintain alignment and ensure your toes, hips and lower abdominals are pressed into the ground

Level 4

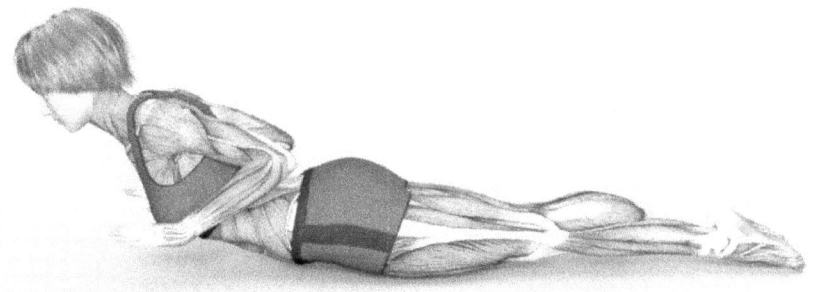

- (Optional) At this point, you can hold the pose and lift the hands away from the floor for a strength challenge
- With palms lifted, pull your shoulders back and down to open the chest

Level 5

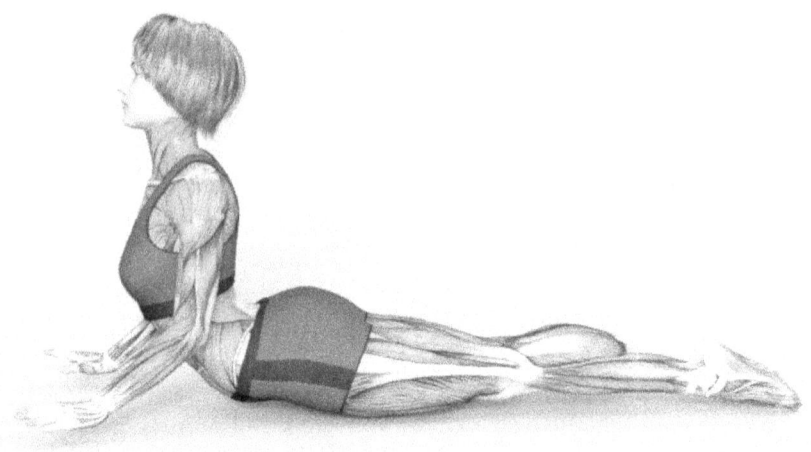

- Maintaining alignment and applied pressure through the palms, hips and feet, extend further into the movement
- Pull your elbows to your sides to eliminate outward flaring of the arms
- Tilt your head backwards to look upwards for an extra stretch through the abdominals

Happy baby

Start position: Supine

Flexibility: 5

This pose is considered a gentle pose, but flexibility through hip opening can be challenged significantly at higher levels.

Strength: 2

Scan for animation

Minimal strength is needed, but there is still an element of core and hip engagement involved

Stability: 1

The stability challenge is minimal in this pose, as we have a large surface area in contact with the ground, and it's a fairly closed position.

Balance: 1

Minimal balance is needed as the body is supported very well in this position.

Muscle Groups Used:

Adductors (inner thighs), hamstrings (rear, upper legs), gluteus maximus and medius (buttocks), psoas and iliacus (hip flexors) core (abdominals, lower back and other stabiliser muscles), biceps and forearms (upper and lower arms).

Extra information: Happy baby pose is used by many as a relaxation pose. It is, however, a great pose for developing flexibility through the hips and hamstrings. Once at level 3 of this pose, we can start to widen the hips further for a greater flexibility challenge in this area.

During the pose, rather than simply holding a static position, it's common to add a slow and controlled sideways rocking, or forward/ backwards movement to add variation to the position. This movement challenges stability and flexibility slightly, but must be controlled and comfortable to perform.

Level 1

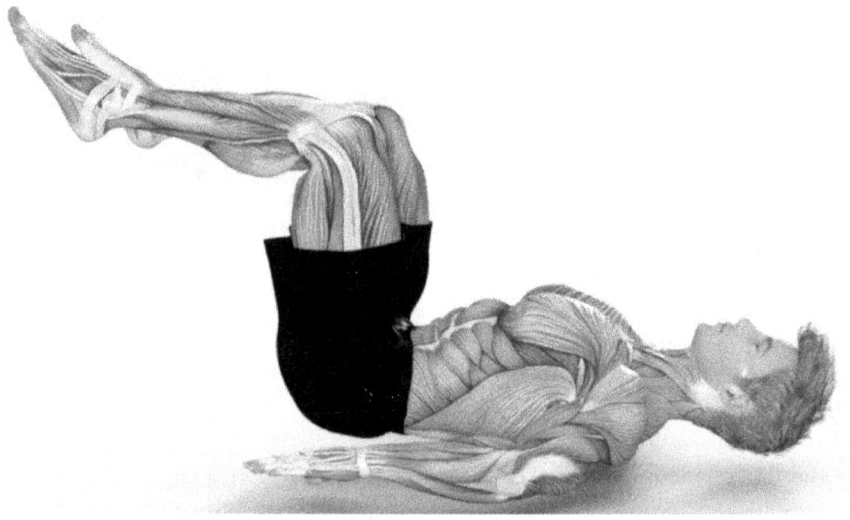

- From the supine starting position, lift your feet away from the floor by bending at the knees and pulling your upper legs towards your chest
- Ensure that you maintain core engagement and alignment through your lower back, especially
- Your back, back of head and shoulders should remain in contact with the ground

Level 2

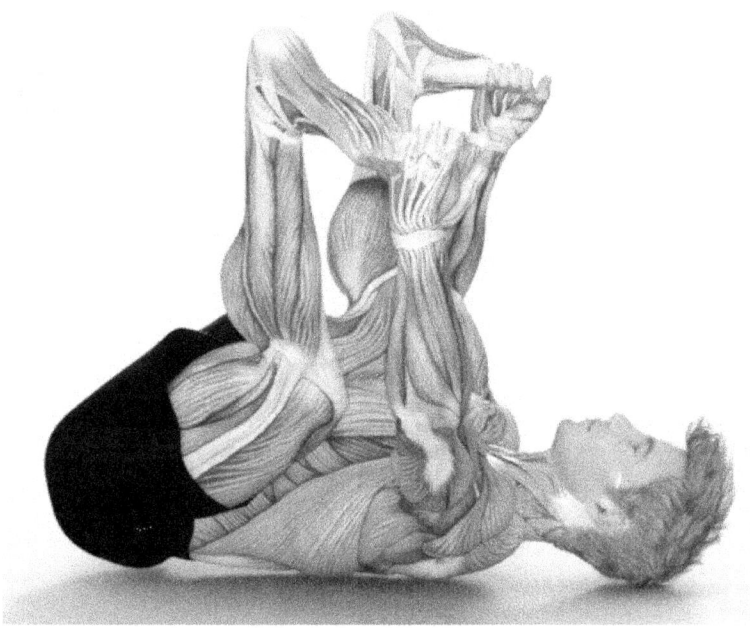

- Reach up with your hands to grasp your big toes with the forefinger, middle finger and thumb of each hand (left hand grasps left big toe, right hand grasps right big toe)
- Continue the knee raise movement until your ankles are above your knees
- Maintain contact with the ground through the back of your head and back
- To increase the movement, gently and under control, bring your upper legs closer to your upper body and out towards the floor

Goddess pose

Scan for animation

Start position: Standing

Strength: 5

Due to the position of this pose, the wide, squatting stance, this pose develops significant strength in the lower body and core.

Flexibility: 4

Develops great flexibility in the lower body through hip opening.

Stability: 4

Stabiliser muscles are challenged from this standing pose. The deeper the squat, the more the challenge.

Balance: 2

Balance is less of an issue for most in this pose as we have a wide foundation to work from.

Muscle Groups Used:

Quadriceps (upper front legs), gluteus maximus and medius (buttocks), adductors (inner thighs), core (abdominals, lower back and other stabiliser muscles), hamstrings (upper, rear legs), soleus and gastrocnemius (lower, rear legs).

Extra information: The goddess pose is a strong, powerful pose that develops strength in the lower body and core. When starting with this pose, prioritise developing the wide stance, glute, and core engagement before lowering into the squat. Maintaining upright alignment during the squatting element of this pose can be a struggle for some, so when it comes to the squat, start shallow and work towards deepening the movement as time goes by.

Level 1

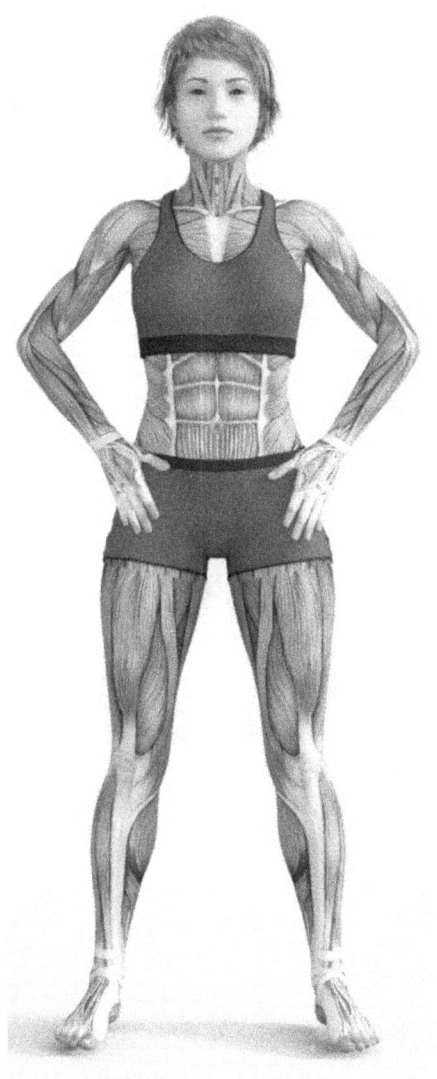

- From the standing start position, place your hands on your hips, keep your legs almost straight, but don't lock your knees
- Position feet about shoulder width apart and distribute your body weight evenly across the soles of your feet

Level 2

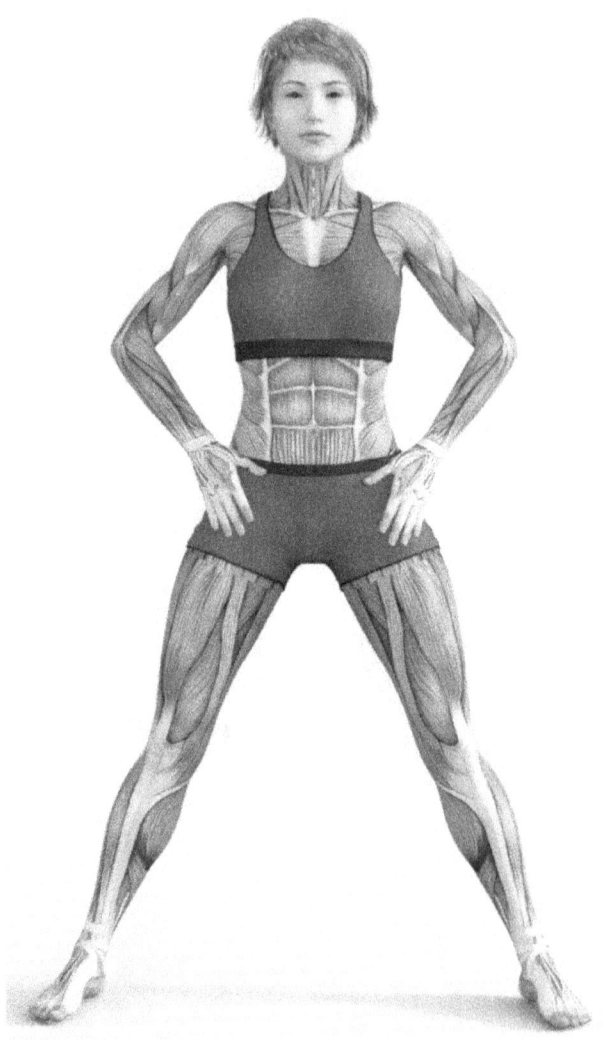

- Take a wider stance with your feet so they are past shoulder width
- Toes can be turned out, up to a forty-five degree angle
- Reassess bodyweight distribution through the feet after widening stance. This should be even throughout the soles

Level 3

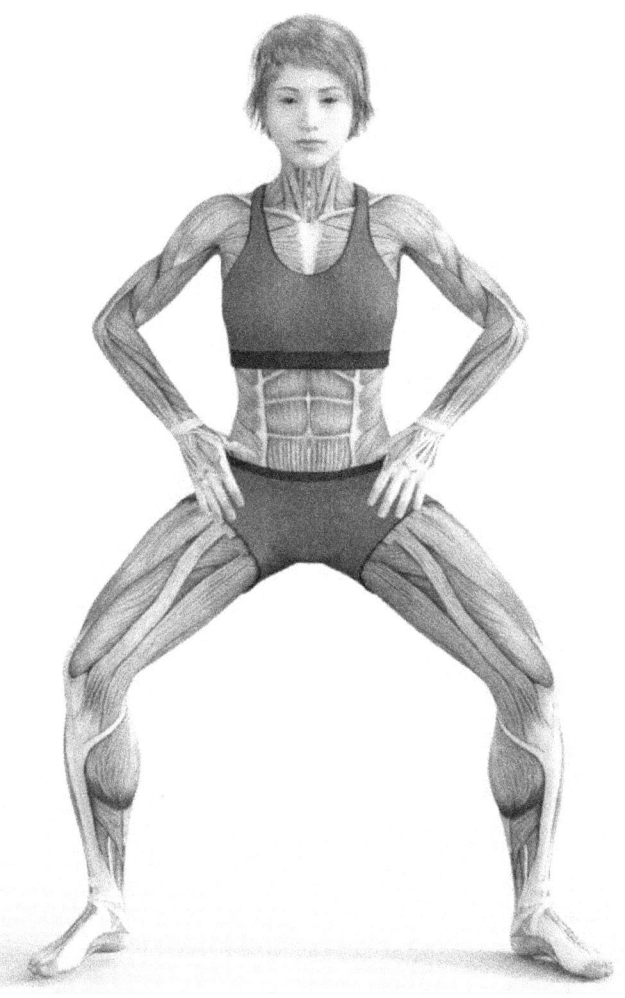

- While maintaining core engagement, alignment through the spine and even weight distribution through the feet, tuck your tailbone by engaging your glutes. This helps to keep your upper body vertical
- Sink into a shallow squat by bending at the knees. Lower to the point that you are comfortable without losing form

Level 4

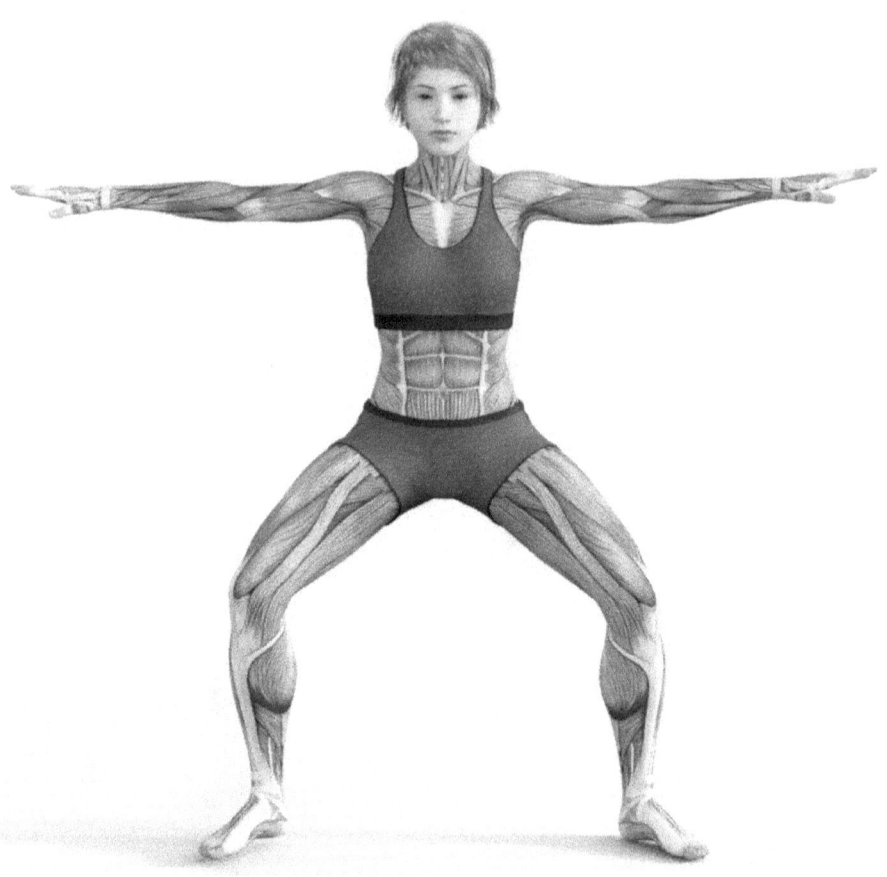

- Maintaining alignment, raise your arms out to your sides until they are parallel with the ground
- Deepen the squat slightly to progress further

Level 5

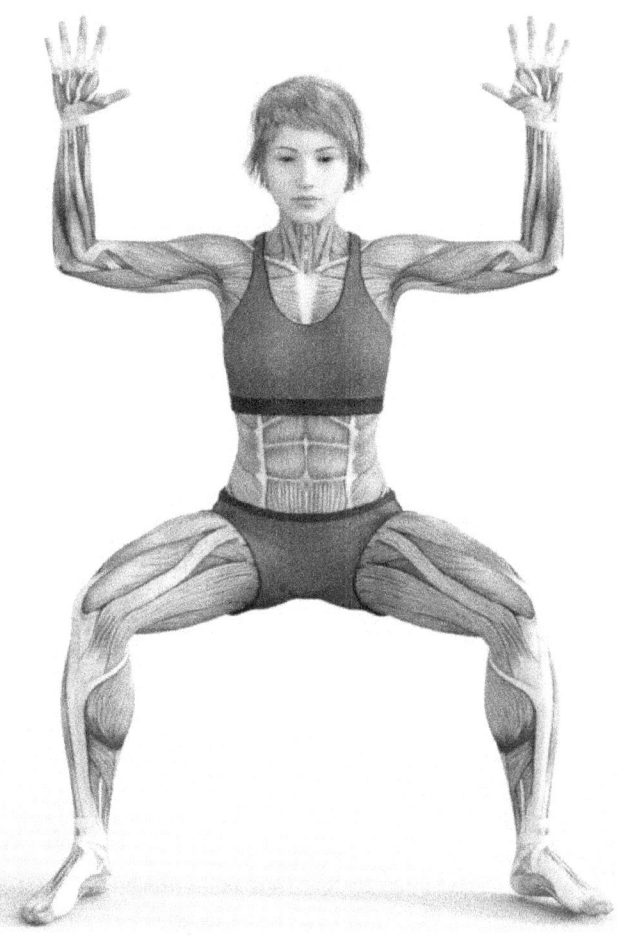

- Continue to deepen the squat while maintaining alignment, core engagement and an even body weight distribution through the planted feet
- Twist the shoulders and bend the elbows to position your arms out to your sides, upper arms parallel to the ground and forearms vertical, palms facing forward

Roll down

Scan for animation

Start position: Standing

Flexibility: 5

Flexibility is the main focus of this pose. The spine is targeted at the first levels and extended to the hamstrings in the latter.

Strength: 3

A moderate strength challenge with this pose as we need controlled muscle engagement of the core and back throughout.

Stability: 3

Stabiliser muscles in the core, legs and back are challenged from this standing pose to a good degree.

Balance: 2

The balance challenge is low as we work from a solid foundation with both feet firmly on the ground.

Muscle Groups Used:

Core (abdominals, lower back and other stabiliser muscles), hamstrings (upper, rear legs), quadriceps (upper front legs), gluteus maximus (buttocks).

Extra information: The roll down is an excellent exercise for developing mobility of the spine, flexibility of the hamstrings and core engagement. When starting out with this pose, the roll down should be slow and controlled, starting with the head and moving incrementally down the spine. There will be a point where the hamstrings start to engage. It's a good idea to be aware of when this happens, as it can be a good measure of progression.

Level 1

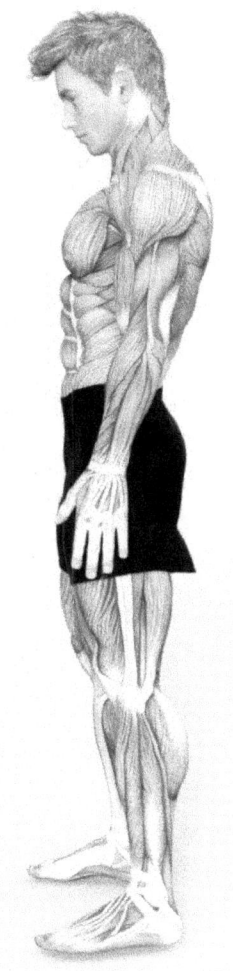

- From the standing start position, slowly tilt your head forward to bring your chin towards your chest

Level 2

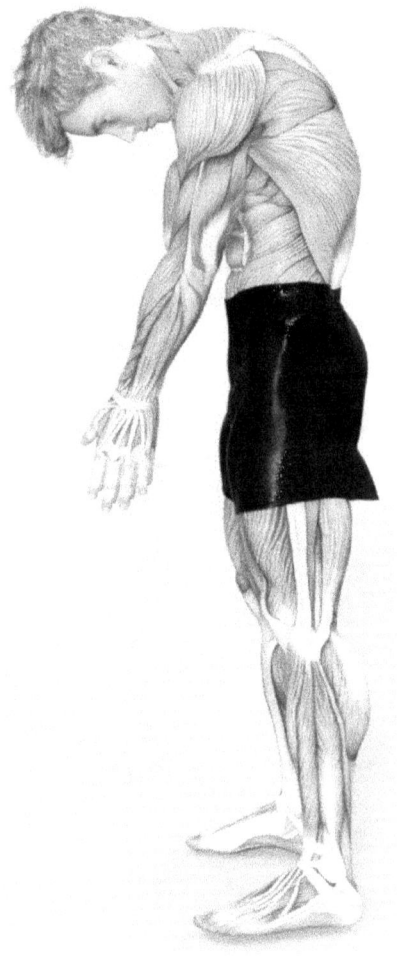

- Slowly continue the head tilt movement by flexing the upper part of your spine forward
- Your arms should naturally start to move forward

Level 3

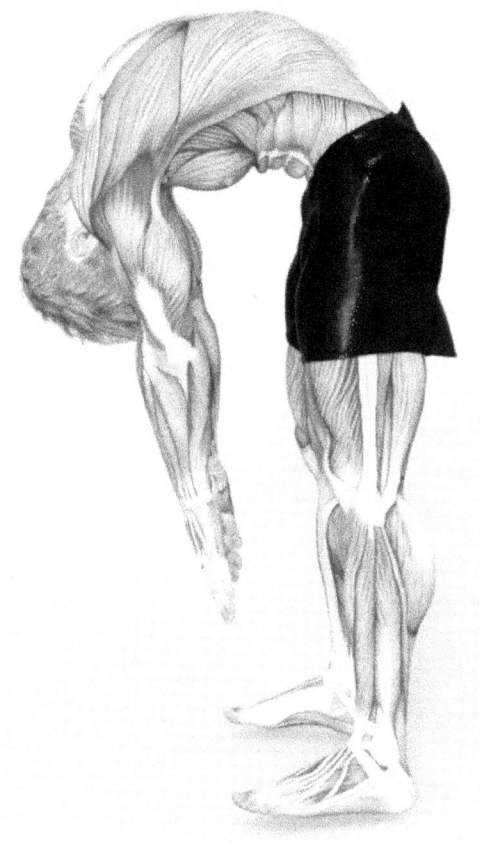

- Slowly continue the forward flexion of your spine down towards your mid and lower back
- You can reach for the floor with your fingertips or keep your arms relaxed in a natural position
- Your knees should stay only slightly bent throughout the movement and chin should stay tucked

Putting it all together

Learning how to perform yoga poses is great, but practicing these poses consistently is the key to progressing through the levels and ultimately reaping the physical, and indeed, psychological rewards.

In all of my fitness guides, I offer a routine card system as an aid to the exercise method. This yoga guide is no different. If we have a goal and a plan, we take away the guesswork each time we settle into a yoga routine, making our sessions efficient, effective, and we can track our progress.

Using the poses from this book, and, indeed, from any other sources you come across, you can create a bespoke yoga plan to fit your specific goals and abilities. Having a routine card set up and in place gives you the opportunity to track your goals and plan for progression.

This is how it works:

ROUTINE #		
YOGA POSE	LEVEL	TIME/REPS/SETS

The top section of the routine card (as shown above) has several fields:

- **Blank row –** This section is reserved for your yoga session name. Fill this in however you like, but I would choose a name that relates to your goal such as "Building strength" or "The balancing act".
- **Routine # -** If you are in for the long haul, the "routine #" row is a great way to track how many times you have progressed, switched up your routine or even changed your goal. Start with the number "1" in here.

- **Yoga pose** – Underneath this heading, you can fill in the poses you plan to perform in each session. You can have up to eleven poses listed in the row below.
- **Level** – This heading is designed to work with the poses described in this guide. In the box adjacent to your chosen pose, write the level number you are planning to perform at.
- **Time/reps/sets** – It's a good idea to have a unit to measure how long you spend on each pose; you could use time, repetitions (reps), or even number of breaths. Fill this in as you see fit. Having a measure like this gives us the opportunity to set goals for further progression.

The lower section of the routine card (pictured below) is a planned yoga session calendar. Fill this in with the days you wish to have yoga sessions. You can plan for seven days and up to six weeks ahead. Simply mark off with a star your yoga session. When you complete that session, put a tick next to it. If you miss it, it's a strike through. This is great for accountability.

WEEKS	MON	TUE	WED	THURS	FRI	SAT	SUN
1							
2							
3							
4							
5							
6							

If you are new to yoga or a beginner to exercise, I'd advise that you fill in no more than three weeks ahead when planning as you may develop quickly, which will give you a chance to update your routine card with further progressions.

Some example routine cards have been created for you to follow or take ideas from. Each of the following routines has a goal, and poses have been selected that are relevant. "Levels" and "time/ reps /sets" are filled in, but bear in mind, if following this yourself that you may work at higher levels or different time, reps or sets ranges, so adjust according to your ability.

Starting out

FUNDAMENTAL YOGA TRAINING		
ROUTINE #		
YOGA POSE	LEVEL	TIME/REPS/SETS
STANDING START POSITION	-	30 SECONDS
FOUR POINT START POSITION	-	30 SECONDS
SEATED START POSITION	-	30 SECONDS
PRONE STARTING POSITION	-	30 SECONDS
SUPINE STARTING POSITION	-	30 SECONDS
HAPPY BABY	1	30 SECONDS

WEEKS	MON	TUE	WED	THURS	FRI	SAT	SUN
1	*		*		*		*
2	*		*		*		*
3	*	*	*	*	*	*	*
4							
5							
6							

This routine card example is a foundation, or beginner session. The main goal here is to develop breathing techniques and awareness of alignment through muscle engagement.

Holding the start positions while concentrating on breathing, body weight distribution and body position can be challenging for some. This routine is not reserved only for total beginners to physical exercise, but those who are starting yoga for the first time can benefit from this too. If you are the type of person that has a busy mind, this routine will give you the opportunity to develop mindfulness, relax, and be in the present.

Thirty seconds are spent in each starting position with the addition of "Happy baby" to finish off with.

This routine can be repeated several times per session. As you can see, each time you run through the entire routine, it should take you about six minutes.

The planned session calendar at the bottom of this chart shows that this is a three week plan with an upgrade to session frequency on the third week.

Yoga for stability and balance

STABILITY & BALANCE YOGA TRAINING

ROUTINE #

YOGA POSE	LEVEL	TIME/REPS/SETS
TREE	5	30 SECS/ 3 SETS
EAGLE	4	30 SECS/ 3 SETS
DANCER	3	30 SECS/ 3 SETS
CHAIR	4	30 SECS/ 3 SETS
FOUR-LIMBED STAFF	2	60 SECS/ 3 SETS
COBRA	4	30 SECS/ 3 SETS

WEEKS	MON	TUE	WED	THURS	FRI	SAT	SUN
1	*	*	*	*	*	*	*
2							
3							
4							
5							
6							

This routine focuses on stability and balance. Each yoga pose on this card is geared towards developing these physical goals.

It's important to remember that each pose that you perform requiring you to create an asymmetrical shape such as standing on one leg poses like "Eagle" and "Dancer" that you repeat the pose to mirror the previous immediately after. So if your left foot is planted in the dancer pose for the first thirty seconds, you then plant your right foot and lift your left leg for the second thirty seconds.

In this particular routine card, under the "Time/reps/sets" heading, each pose is performed for "30 seconds" and is repeated "3 times". If you are following this as it is set out and this is too much, simply reduce the sets.

Under the heading "Level", there is a fairly big range on this example. This is realistic, as everyone will have their strengths and weaknesses through different poses. It's important that you work within your range making small adjustments towards progression in each pose, so you may have to switch these up.

The session calendar at the bottom of the routine card shows that this is a daily session for the first week, signalling that this will be reviewed and possibly updated at the start of the next week.

Flexibility

FLEXIBILITY YOGA TRAINING		

ROUTINE #		

YOGA POSE	LEVEL	TIME/REPS/SETS
ROLL DOWN	2	30 SECS/ 3 SETS
HAPPY BABY	2	30 SECS/ 3 SETS
FORWARD FOLD	1	30 SECS/ 3 SETS
COBRA	3	30 SECS/ 3 SETS
SUPINE STARTING POSITION	-	60 SECONDS

WEEKS	MON	TUE	WED	THURS	FRI	SAT	SUN
1	*	*	*	*	*	*	*
2							
3							
4							
5							
6							

This routine card is focused on flexibility through the back and legs. Each exercise is performed for thirty seconds and three times. After each thirty-second pose, there is a brief return to the starting position before repeating the pose for another thirty seconds.

The last exercise is a sixty-second hold of the supine starting position to finish the session. This last pose can be used for developing mindfulness.

The planned weekly session calendar shows that this is a one week, daily routine that will possibly be updated before the start of the next week.

Yoga for strength

STRENGTH YOGA TRAINING

ROUTINE #

YOGA POSE	LEVEL	TIME/REPS/SETS
WARRIOR	4	30 SECS/ 3 SETS
CHAIR	3	30 SECS/ 3 SETS
GODDESS	4	30 SECS/ 3 SETS
BRIDGE	2	30 SECS/ 3 SETS
FOUR-LIMBED STAFF	2	60 SECS/ 3 SETS
HAPPY BABY	2	60 SECONDS

WEEKS	MON	TUE	WED	THURS	FRI	SAT	SUN
1	*	*	*	*	*	*	*
2							
3							
4							
5							
6							

The focus of this routine card is on strength development. Each yoga pose in this routine is a strong one, bar the last (happy baby).

As usual, poses like "warrior" which position your body asymmetrically should be mirrored immediately after a thirty-second hold of the position has been completed; if your left foot is facing forward on the first thirty-second hold, your right foot faces forward on the next thirty-second hold.

Some levels on this particular routine card are higher on some poses than others, but this will be dictated by your current development level, so edit this if you wish to follow this example routine.

The pose "happy baby" has been added as the last pose on this routine to alleviate any tension in the legs and as a relaxation aid.

All rounder

ALL ROUNDER YOGA TRAINING

ROUTINE #

YOGA POSE	LEVEL	TIME/REPS/SETS
GODDESS	5	30 SECS/ 3 SETS
WARRIOR	4	30 SECS/ 3 SETS
TREE	4	30 SECS/ 3 SETS
DANCER	4	30 SECS/ 3 SETS
FOUR-LIMBED STAFF	2	60 SECS/ 3 SETS
FORWARD FOLD	4	30 SECS/ 3 SETS
COBRA	5	30 SECS/ 3 SETS

WEEKS	MON	TUE	WED	THURS	FRI	SAT	SUN
1	*	*	*	*	*	*	*
2							
3							
4							
5							
6							

This routine card draws from all four pillars of yoga fitness mentioned in this book; strength, flexibility, stability and balance. This is a well-rounded routine that can be used for the long term.

The levels listed here are on the higher end of the scale, but it can be adapted to fit anyone's current ability.

As per the other routines, this has several poses listed that position the body asymmetrically, so each pose that does this (warrior and tree) should be mirrored and repeated after each thirty-second hold.

The sets and reps can also be adapted to fit your needs if you wish to follow this routine as it is set out.

The split

SPLIT		
ROUTINE #		
A YOGA POSE	LEVEL	TIME/REPS/SETS
GODDESS	5	30 SECS/ 3 SETS
WARRIOR	4	30 SECS/ 3 SETS
TREE	4	30 SECS/ 3 SETS
DANCER	4	30 SECS/ 3 SETS
FOUR-LIMBED STAFF	2	60 SECS/ 3 SETS
FORWARD FOLD	4	30 SECS/ 3 SETS
COBRA	5	30 SECS/ 3 SETS
B YOGA POSE	LEVEL	TIME/REPS/SETS
ROLL DOWN	2	30 SECS/ 3 SETS
HAPPY BABY	2	30 SECS/ 3 SETS
FORWARD FOLD	1	30 SECS/ 3 SETS
COBRA	3	30 SECS/ 3 SETS
SUPINE STARTING POSITION	-	60 SECONDS

WEEKS	MON	TUE	WED	THURS	FRI	SAT	SUN
1	A	B	REST	A	B	REST	REST
2	A	B	REST	A	B	REST	REST
3	A	B	REST	A	B	A	B
4							
5							
6							

For those who like to plan ahead, have multiple goals and would like a more diverse yoga routine, a split plan can be used. This example takes the yoga routine focused on strength and the flexibility routine and merges them into a single card.

In the "yoga pose" column heading, there is now either "A" or "B". In this case "A" indicates the strength routine and the "B" indicates the flexibility routine.

During a week, the routines are performed successively; "A" (strength yoga session on Monday), "B" (flexibility yoga session on Tuesday) and so on. There are rest days added to plan for days with no session, but these can be planned according to your plans, goals, and development.

A split routine can be used for any type of goal. For example, it may be that you would like an all-round yoga session with an extra day to work on flexibility if you would like to put a heavier focus on flexibility.

Although this type of planning may seem to take a bit of the "freedom" associated with yoga away, and add rigidity to it, it's a great tool to use for tracking progression and for accountability if you are serious about the physical results of yoga workouts.

Chair yoga poses

I have written several other exercise guides that focus on specific training methods. There is something for everyone. One such guide was for those who are looking to exercise from a seated position on a chair. Chair workouts could be used for many reasons, and although this seems limiting, it's not as limiting as some may think.

In my book titled "Chair workouts", there are several training methods outlined, along with illustrated descriptions of exercises that use bodyweight, resistance bands and other functional movement methods. There is also a section on chair yoga.

The following pages on chair yoga poses are taken from this guide. If you are planning to create your own yoga routine using the blank routine cards provided in this book, and would like a seated option, these might be worth considering.

If you would also like to learn more about the possibilities of chair exercise, have a look at this one. Maybe you'd like to try adding some exercise bands to a workout or would like to develop strength in certain areas with bodyweight movements? I'll look forward to seeing you again!

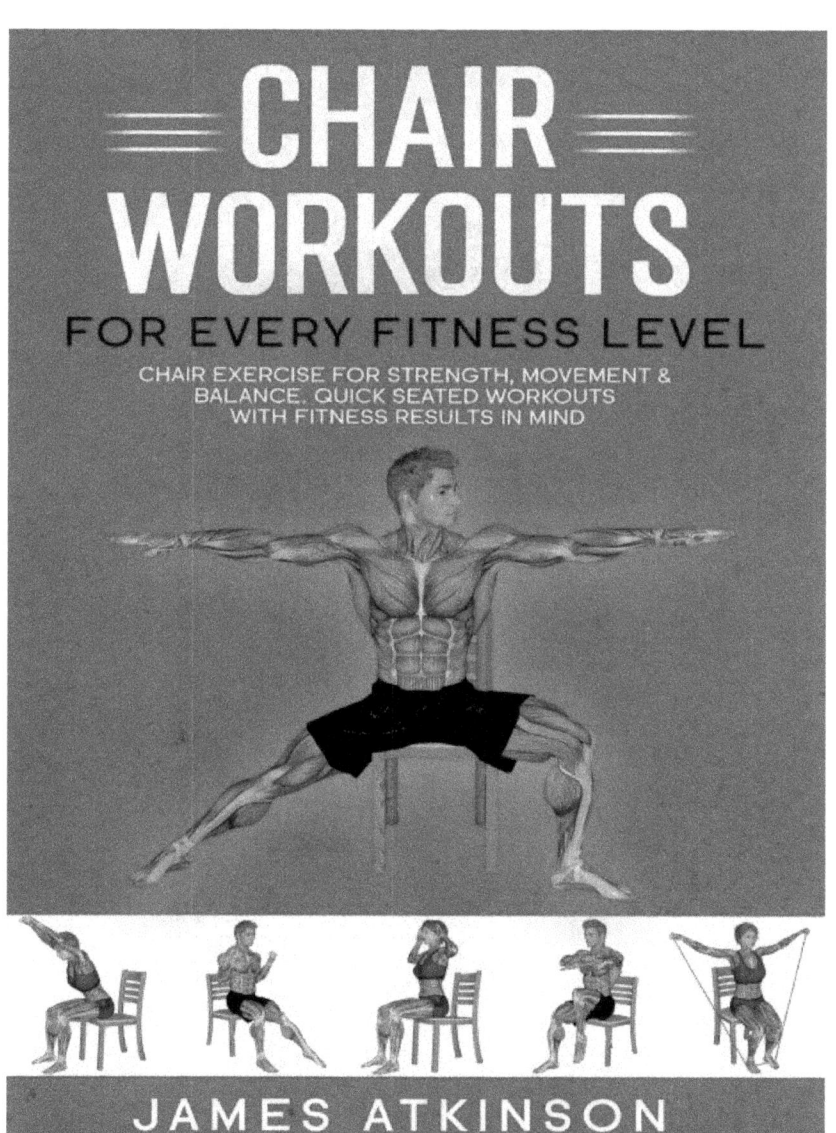

Pigeon pose

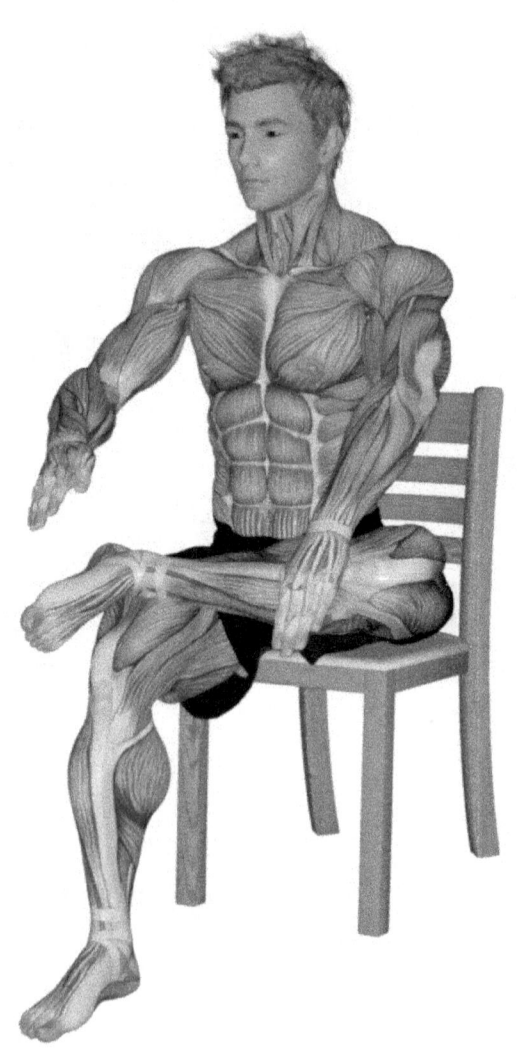

- From the default position, bring your left leg off the floor and bend at the knee
- Keep your right foot planted firmly on the floor
- Twist your hip to rest on the outside of your left ankle just above your right knee
- Keep your back flat and upper body aligned as per the default position
- Use your right hand to hold your left ankle in place if you need to
- (Optional) Apply a small amount of pressure to your left knee to increase the range of movement
- Hold for your planned time before slowly reversing the movement back to the default position before repeating on the opposite leg

If the knee of your working leg points up at an angle, this is very common and not a problem. Hold the position only to the point that you are comfortable with. You can work towards lowering the knee over time.

Seated tree

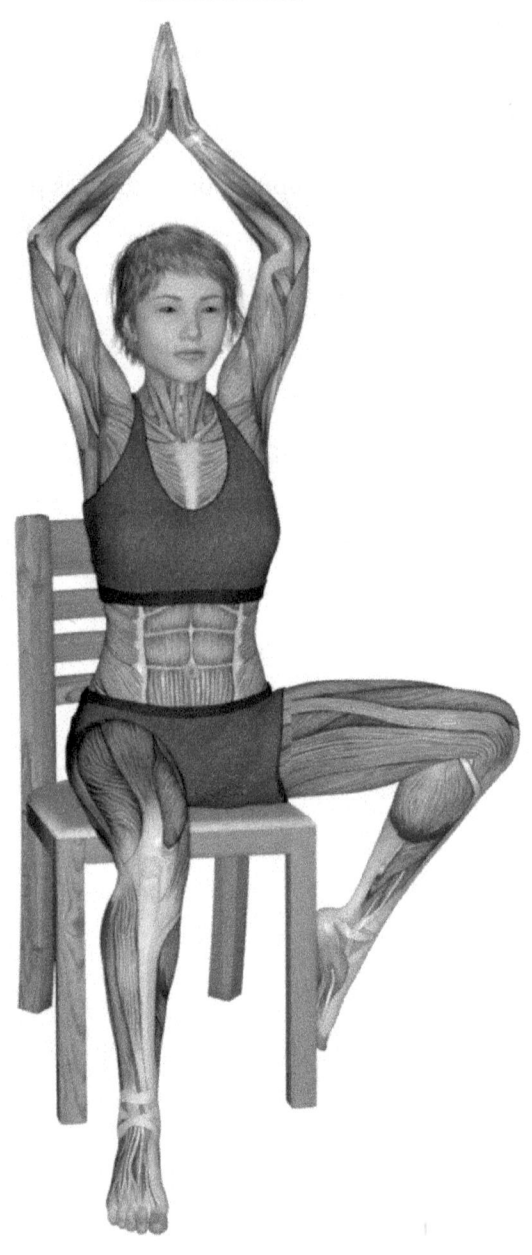

- From the default position, lift your left leg away from the floor by bending at the knee
- Rotate your left hip and bend your left ankle to place the sole of your left foot on the side of the left chair leg
- Ensure that your hips and torso remain forward, facing
- Keep your right foot planted firmly on the floor
- Engage your abdominals and core
- Raise both arms directly above your head
- Turn your palms inwards and place them together, fingers pointing directly up
- Hold for your planned time before returning to the default position
- Rebuild the pose with the opposite leg and repeat the build of your upper body to ensure both hips benefit from the same intensity

Half moon

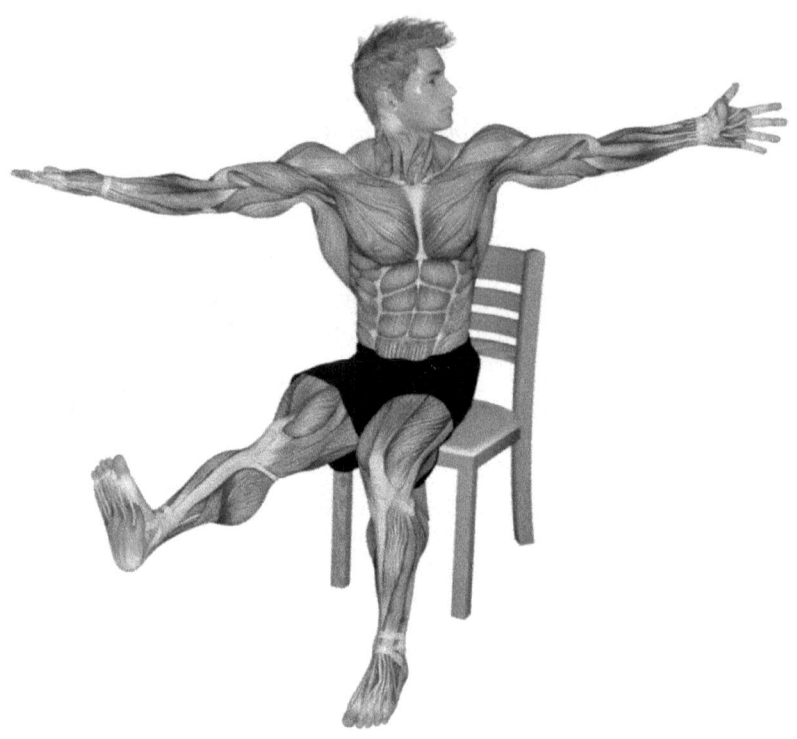

- From the default position, straighten your right leg by bending at the knee
- Keep your hips facing forward and abdominals and core engaged
- Raise both arms out to your sides so they are parallel with the floor
- Twist your right wrist so your palm is facing upwards
- Twist your left wrist so your palm is facing forward
- From this position, twist your torso to the left
- Once your torso twist has reached its maximum range of motion, turn your head to look directly down your left arm

- Hold this position for your planned time before returning to the default position and rebuilding with the opposite leg and twisting in the opposite direction

A couple of things to be aware of on this one: Make sure your straight leg doesn't drop. Be aware of your arm positioning; it's common to lose focus on your "palm up" arm as this is behind your head. It can drift forward or drop. Finally, be aware of your back and hip positioning when building the position and when holding; it's easy to round the back and rotate the hips, especially during the torso twist.

Camel

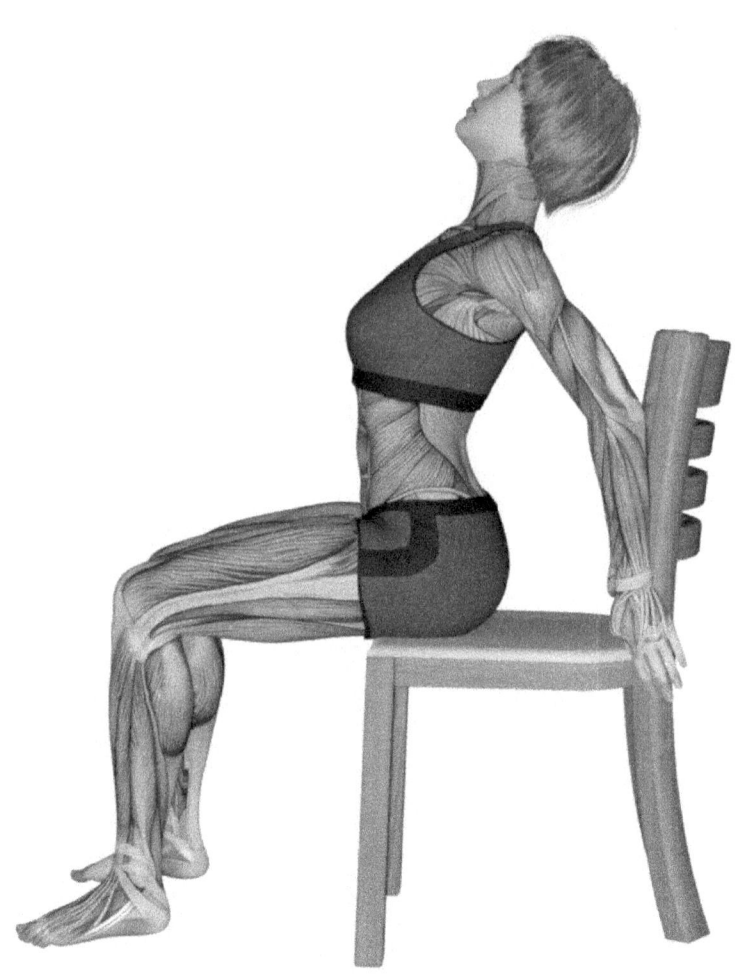

- Set up the default position so that your glutes are slightly further forward on the chair than normal. You will need the extra space behind you
- While maintaining your back alignment, push your arms backwards so you are able to grip the rear of the seat or the backrest of the chair
- Your palms should be facing inwards and arms straight or with a slight bend at the elbows
- As you exhale, push your chest up and forwards
- Continue this movement by pulling your shoulders back and down
- Once you have reached the limit of your range of motion in this movement, hold the position
- Once this position is stable, tilt your head to look upwards

Forward fold & prayer

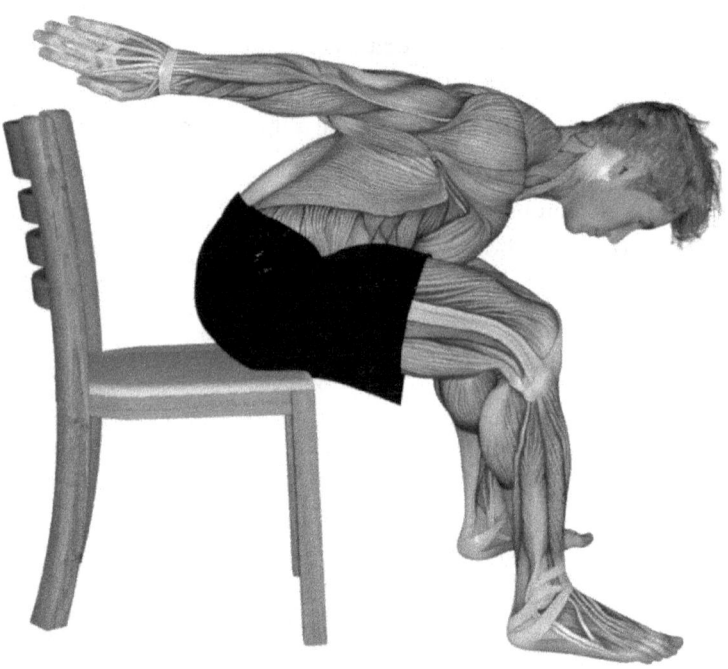

- Set up in the default position as usual, but position your feet on the floor slightly wider than hip width apart
- As you exhale, hinge at the hips to bring your upper body towards your upper legs
- Ensure you do not round the rest of your back when moving into this position and keep your head and neck in a neutral position
- Once you have reached your maximum range of movement with the forward fold, with straight arms, rotate your shoulders to bring your arms back and behind your torso, palms facing inwards
- At this point, you can either rest your fingertips on the backrest or pull your shoulders closer together to clasp the fingers of both hands together
- Hold this position for your planned timeframe and slowly reverse the process to return to the default position

This pose is great developing strength and mobility in the shoulders, lower back and core. As we can't see our arm position, it's common to let them bend more than we would like at the elbows, so this is something to be aware of. Also, this is a fairly tricky pose for a lot of people with lower back and shoulder issues, so the range of movement may differ fairly drastically from the diagram for some. Time and consistency with the exercise will always help.

Twist & prayer

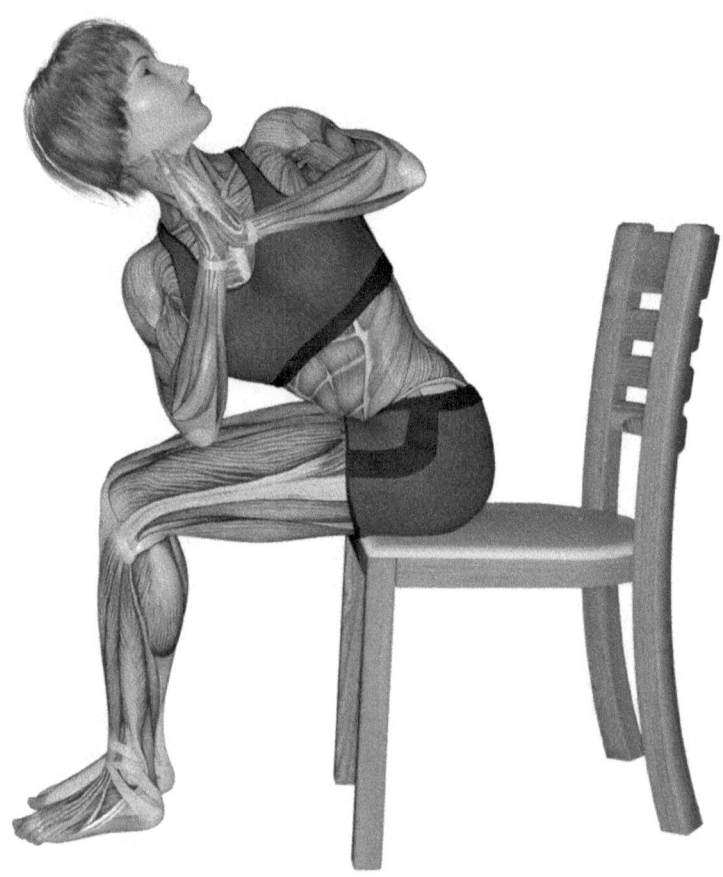

- Set up in the default position, but plant your feet on the floor close together. The insides of your feet, knees and upper legs should be touching each other
- From this position, twist at your waist towards your left-hand side until you reach your maximum range of movement

- Bring your palms into a prayer position (palms touching, fingers pointed upwards) close to your body and in line with your upper chest
- Turn your head to look at your left shoulder
- You can choose to hold the position at this point
- To develop the movement further, bend at the waist to drop your right elbow towards your left knee
- To increase shoulder mobility from here, shift your palms towards your left shoulder by pushing your right shoulder forward and left shoulder backwards
- Once you have held your chosen variation of this position, slowly return to the default position and repeat on the other side

Your yoga routine

The routines set out in this book can be followed directly, but not everyone is at the same stage of yoga development or, indeed, has the same goals for yoga sessions. For this reason, I think it's important that we ask ourselves what we would like to get from these sessions and plan from there.

Some may want to use yoga as a mindfulness tool and plan to spend full sessions practicing breathing and muscle awareness, some may want to focus on exclusively developing either flexibility, stability, strength or balance, while others would like a session that encompasses all the above. It may be that some people want to develop to the highest levels of a pose set out in this guide, whereas others are happy with the benefits of a lower level.

There are many scenarios, so blank yoga routine cards have been added at the end of this guide for you to copy and use to adapt to your personal circumstance and yoga goals.

As always, if you would like PDF copies of these, please give me a shout at:

Admin@yourfitnesssuccess.com

I'll send them over.

I hope this guide has been helpful. I would like to thank you for your purchase and wish you all the best with your yoga sessions.

Namaste

Jim (James Atkinson)

Video course

If you found this guide helpful and you are a beginner to weight loss and exercise, I have something that might help you!

My genuine passion as a fitness professional is helping the beginner earn their first actual results. This stage of the journey can be truly life changing. I have always empathised with the feeling of not being able to get where we want to be. I also know the feeling of overwhelm when there's too much information on a subject. So I created a video course that any beginner can follow from their own home. Just press the play button and we both train together!

We will work on a weekly basis, the first week is really an important week where we lay the foundations, we'll sit down and start planning for success, well find our motivation, get specific about our goals, I always advise making these goals ambitious because we can all achieve more than we think we can!

Week 1 through to week 6 is where we hit our home workouts! Each week is more progressive than the last. We build on our training from the previous week by tweaking the exercise choices, adding intensity and further challenging ourselves. Some people develop quicker and can move from week to week seamlessly, but the beauty of this course is that if you find a week a bit too challenging, you can repeat the previous week. Everyone moves at a different pace, so it's no problem!

So if this sounds like something you are interested in, please check out the video testimonials, check out the sample videos and you can even start the course for free!

It would be great to see you over at:

YourFitnessSuccess.com

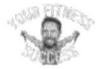

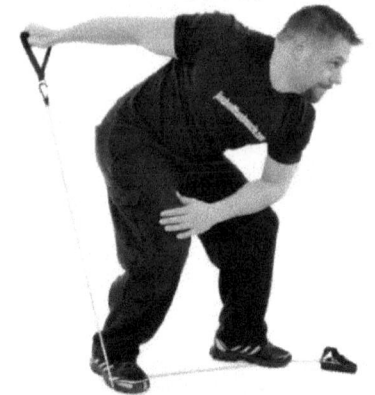

Online Home Workout Courses

Fitness results you can count on!

No gimmicks, no fads, just real advice with results in mind.

Let's do this!

START THE COURSE FOR FREE

What do others think about this course?

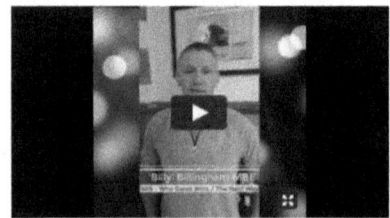
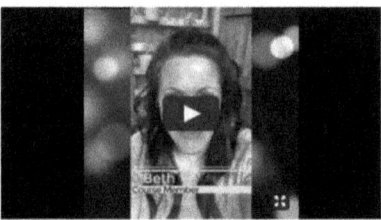

"Far more than your usual fitness video training! This is a serious, progressive exercise course!"

You can start the course right now for free and grab some freebies that might help with your fitness goals at the same time! I'll see you there!

https://yourfitnesssuccess.com/all-the-freebiees/

Blank routine cards

ROUTINE #	

YOGA POSE	LEVEL	TIME/REPS/SETS

WEEKS	MON	TUE	WED	THURS	FRI	SAT	SUN
1							
2							
3							
4							
5							
6							

ROUTINE #	

YOGA POSE	LEVEL	TIME/REPS/SETS

WEEKS	MON	TUE	WED	THURS	FRI	SAT	SUN
1							
2							
3							
4							
5							
6							

ROUTINE #	

YOGA POSE	LEVEL	TIME/REPS/SETS

WEEKS	MON	TUE	WED	THURS	FRI	SAT	SUN
1							
2							
3							
4							
5							
6							

SPLIT		
ROUTINE #		

A	YOGA POSE	LEVEL	TIME/REPS/SETS

B	YOGA POSE	LEVEL	TIME/REPS/SETS

WEEKS	MON	TUE	WED	THURS	FRI	SAT	SUN
1							
2							
3							
4							
5							
6							

SPLIT		
ROUTINE #		

A	YOGA POSE	LEVEL	TIME/REPS/SETS

B	YOGA POSE	LEVEL	TIME/REPS/SETS

WEEKS	MON	TUE	WED	THURS	FRI	SAT	SUN
1							
2							
3							
4							
5							
6							

	SPLIT		
ROUTINE #			

A	YOGA POSE	LEVEL	TIME/REPS/SETS

B	YOGA POSE	LEVEL	TIME/REPS/SETS

WEEKS	MON	TUE	WED	THURS	FRI	SAT	SUN
1							
2							
3							
4							
5							
6							

Also by James Atkinson

Scan below for more guides like this

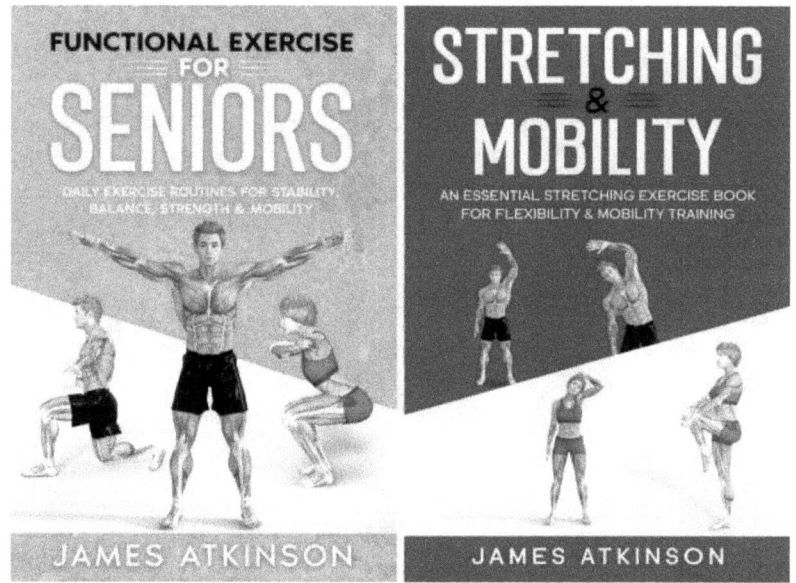

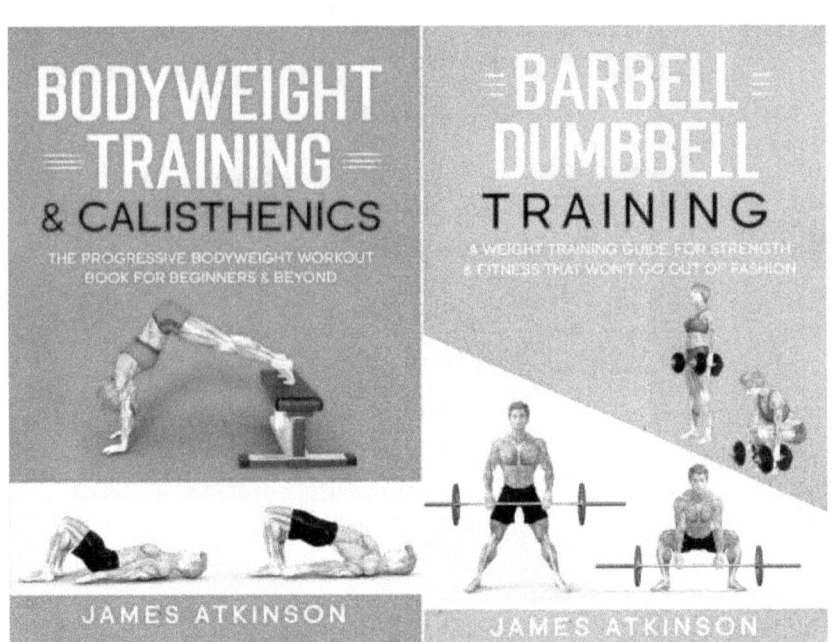
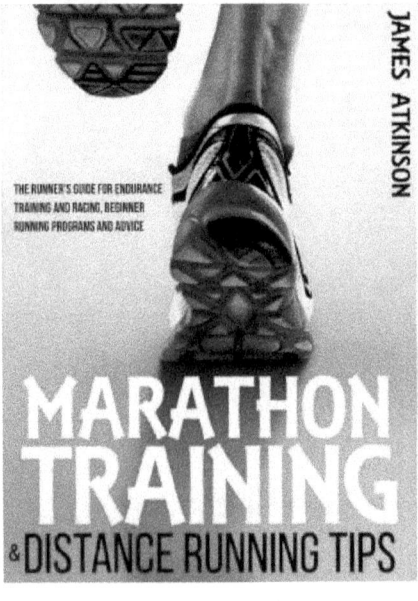
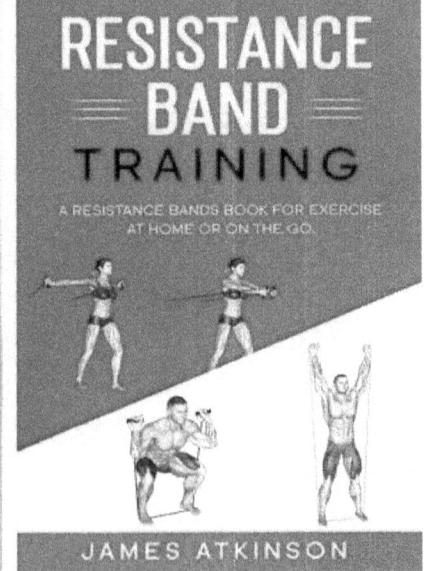

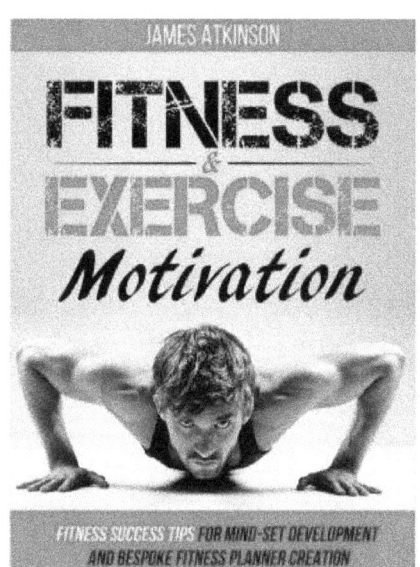
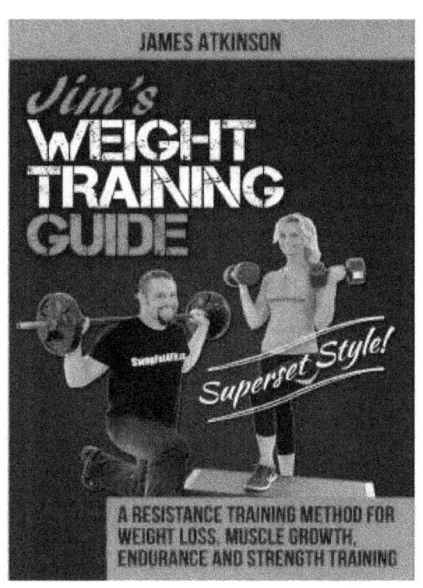
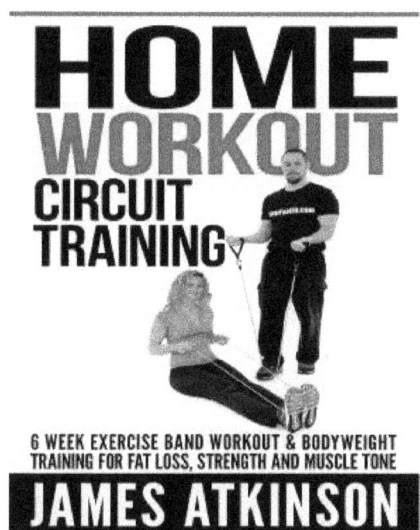
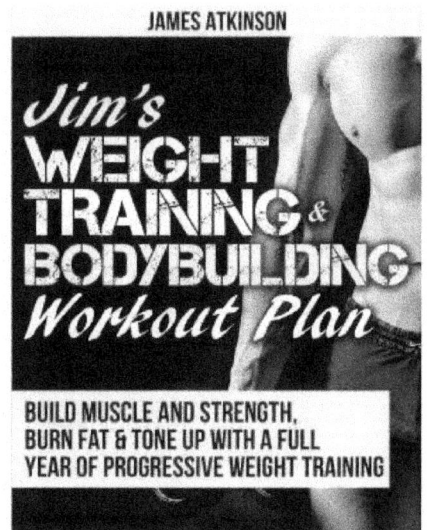

YOURFITNESSSUCCESS.COM

PAPERBACK EDITION

PUBLISHED BY: JBA Publishing

http://www.yourfitnesssuccess.com

admin@yourfitnesssuccess.com

Yoga For Strength And Stability

Copyright © 2025 by James Atkinson

All Rights Reserved.

No part of this book may be reproduced or transmitted in any form or by any means, electronic, mechanical, photocopying, recording, or otherwise, without the prior written permission of James Atkinson, except for brief quotations in critical reviews or articles.

Requests for permission to make copies of any part of this book should be submitted to James Atkinson at admin@yourfitnesssuccess.com

DISCLAIMER

Although the author and publisher have made every effort to ensure that the information contained in this book was accurate at the time of release, the author and publisher do not assume and hereby disclaim any liability to any party for any loss, damage, or disruption caused by errors or omissions in this book, whether such errors or omissions result from negligence, accident, or any other cause.

First published in 2025

www.ingramcontent.com/pod-product-compliance
Lightning Source LLC
Chambersburg PA
CBHW071714020426
42333CB00017B/2273